Your Modeling Career

You Don't Have to Be a Supermodel to Succeed

~

Debbie and Skip Press

D1422266

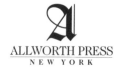

ALLWORTH PRESS
NEW YORK

05 04 03 02   5   4   3   2

Published by Allworth Press
An imprint of Allworth Communications
10 East 23rd Street, New York, NY 10010

Cover design by Douglas Design Associates, New York, NY

Page composition/typography by Sharp Des!gns, Lansing, MI

ISBN: 1–58115–045–8

LIBRARY OF CONGRESS CATALOGING–IN PUBLICATION DATA

Press, Skip, 1950 –
Your modeling career: you don't have to be a supermodel to succeed / Skip and Debbie Press.
        p. cm.
Includes index.
ISBN 1–58115–045–8 (pbk.)
  1. Models (Persons)--Vocational guidance. I. Press, Debbie. II. Title.

HD8039.M77P74 2000
746.9'2'02373--dc21   00–024650

Printed in Canada

Table of Contents

Acknowledgements .... *vii*

Foreword *by Skip Press* .... *ix*

Introduction *by Debbie Press* .... *xi*

1   The World of Modeling *1*
Where You Need to Live • It All Begins at Home • The Ever–
Changing Business • Do You Have "The Look"? • Your Future in
Modeling

2   The Different Types of Modeling *9*
Print Work • Parts or Specialty Work • Glamour Modeling •
Runway • Fit Modeling • Showroom Modeling • Promotional
Modeling • Television and Film Work

3   Model Types: Beyond Beautiful **33**
Petites • Full–Figure or Large–Size Models • Males • Juniors •
Children • Mature Models • Characters

4   Do You Have What It Takes? **41**
What Does It Take Physically? • Beyond Beauty

5   Creating Your Image **57**
Basic Skin Care • Body Care • Posture • Nail Care • Feet •
Dental Care • Makeup • Hair Care • Overall Health •
Developing Your Own Style

6   Finding the Right Agency **75**
Small–Town Realities • Average–Size Cities Outside the Major
Markets • Major Markets • Tips for Finding an Agency •
Interview Questions • Unknown Agencies

7   All About Agencies **85**
What Does a Modeling Agency Do? • Model Management
Companies • Agency Professionals • The Test Board • Agencies
and Housing • Travel and Relocation • The Contract •
Promotion • Finding New Models • Money Matters

8   Building Your Portfolio **97**
Posing • Makeup for the Camera • A New You? • Your
Portfolio • Testings • Model Release

9   Congratulations! You Booked the Job! **115**
Your First Booking • Rates and Scheduling • Booking Form •
More about Bookings • Voucher Forms • Things You Will Need •
Professionalism • Keeping Your Balance

10   Avoiding the Dark Side of the Business **127**
Listen to Your Instincts • Advertisements • High Salaries •
Flexible Schedules • Modeling Scouts • Examining Your

Potential • Investigating an Agency • Money in Advance •
Unprofessional Behavior • Substance Abuse • Contracts •
Conventions • Schools • Federal Trade Commission

11 *Travel and Relocation* **141**
Relocating to New York • Learning about New York • Hotels •
Residences • International Travel • Your Passport • Money,
Traveler's Checks, and Foreign Currency

12 *International Modeling* **149**
Australia • England • France • Germany • Greece • Italy •
Japan • Scandinavia • Spain • Switzerland

13 *Modeling and the Internet* **157**
Online Agencies • Investigating Scams • Forums and Chat Sites •
Sleazy Sites • Cyber Models • Finding Photographers on the Web

14 *The Business Basics* **167**
Taxes • The Model's Guild • Making Ends Meet • Preparing and
Living within a Budget • Savings • Investing in Your Career •
Model Contracts

15 *Careers in Fashion and Related Industries* **175**
Acting • Agent/Booker • Photographer • Fashion Designer •
Fashion Writers and Editors for Magazines and Trades • Fashion
Stylist • Makeup Artist • Hairstylist • Stylist • Broadcasting •
Artist's Representative/Agent • Advertising • Public Relations •
Set Designer

16 *Advice for Concerned Parents* **183**
Teens in the Adult Market • A Look at Agencies • Starting Out •
Trusting Your Teenage Model • Managing Your Young Model's
Career • Education • Travel • Coping with Change • Money
Management • Homesickness • Final Thoughts on Teens and
Modeling • From Babies to Young Teens

17   Training **195**
Role–Model School • Finding a Modeling School

18   Conventions and Contests **201**
Model Search America • Modeling Association of America Inter-
national, Inc. • New York Model Contracts • A Word about Rip–Off
Conventions

19   The Agencies **207**
United States • International

20   Resources **225**
Books • Videos • Makeup Products/Lessons • Modeling Supplies
and Books • Composite Cards and Digital Services • Web Sites

Contributing Photographers and Artists **237**

Glossary of Modeling and Related Terms **245**

Index **249**

Acknowledgements

$\mathcal{D}$eb and Skip Press would like to dedicate this book to those who do their best to inspire others to achieve their dreams.

A very special thanks to Tad Crawford and Allworth Press, for making this book possible, and to two superb editors, Nicole Potter and Jamie Kijowski, with a deeply grateful indebtedness to world-renowned writer Michael Sedge for the introduction.

Deb would like to personally thank those who offered encouragement, enthusiasm, and inspiration in the "modeling days" and during the process of writing this book.

First and foremost, Michele August, president of 212 Artist Representatives, for being a great friend, offering a wealth of advice and expertise, sweating through the research and writing processes, and for introducing me to top professionals in the world of fashion.

To those professionals who gave their time and knowledge: Monique

Pilard, president, Elite Model Management; Wendy Rose, Ford Models; Susan Georget and Fran Palumbo, Wilhelmina Models; Kwok Kan Chan, Marilyn; Michelle Thomas, Madison; Charles Short, Aline Souliers Management; David Vando, Models Mart; Karl Rudisill, president of DICE; Gideon Lewin, photographer; F. David Mogull, president Model Search America; Linda Bennett, New York Model Contracts; photographer Pascal Preti; Carole Treuhaft; Karen Lee, Models Stephanie Averill, Laura Gens, Ellen Sirot, Shannon Marie Codner, Luria Petrucci, Joanna Marie, Leslie Adair, Danielle Peterson, Brian White; Kristina Proulx; Michele Persinger; photographers Karim Ramiz, Johnny Olsen, Andrew Richard, D. Brian Nelson, and John Hall; make-up artists Sherrie Long and Carole Weamer; Molly Peterson of MJP Artists; and the photographers and artists who contributed their time and allowed their wonderful art and images to become a part of this book.

To Martin Snaric for showing me the power of having a burning desire to succeed; John Blankenship for introducing me to the world of photography and encouraging me to "go for it"; colleagues of past and present who offered support and encouragement, primarily Lenore Marta, Kristy Sanchez, Jo Anne Klein, John McElwain, Janice Neenan, Maryanne Bardin, Joanne Julian, Joan Fry, and Lila Suda.

To my supportive family (Mike, Francie, Julie, and Les) for always being there—especially in those homesick modeling days—and to my father, Jarrell Hartsog, who has never failed to be right there when needed, with the exact, right words to say.

To my two beautiful children, Haley and Holly, for putting up with eating at McDonald's and ordering pizza (my, what a sacrifice!) during the writing of this book.

Most of all, my heartfelt thanks to my husband and cowriter, Skip Press, without whom this book would not exist. I will always remember your faith in me, the encouragement you offered, your amazing editing expertise, and this special opportunity to create a book and fulfill a dream.

∽

Foreword

*T*he human form has been an object of admiration since the beginning of time, yet physical beauty is often subjective. Every time the fashion industry has a favorite look–a waifish, forlorn, gamine quality, perhaps–some new model comes along who has a mole or beauty mark that she refuses to remove, or she actually smiles (gasp!) as the photographer takes her picture. Tastes change all the time.

No matter what your physical attributes or gender, there may be a place for you in front of the camera. You may find, however, that you prefer a place behind the camera, or in some other part of the business.

My wife, Debra Press, discovered that writing a book about a profession at which she succeeded–one that she began "late," as far as models go, and at which no one expected her to succeed–gave her as much satisfaction as strutting down a runway or rushing along hot New York streets to make it to a "go-see" (appointment) in time. In writing, she doesn't have to have her hair and makeup perfect, and she doesn't ruin

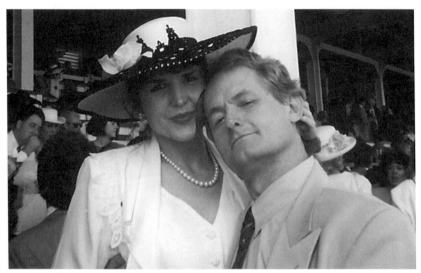

Debbie and Skip Press. Photo by Chris Patton.

yet another pair of high heels in hot summer asphalt, stepping across a Manhattan pothole.

Of course, she and I have spent a good deal of time in our lives doing things that people told us were impossible. We've countered the type of opposition that you may come up against if you announce to your family and friends one day that you would like to be a successful model. If it's in your heart, if you have the physical qualifications, and if you have that special indefinable quality known as "the camera loves you," don't listen to anyone who doesn't help you reach your dream.

This book is a dream of sorts for Debbie in that, via these pages, she is able to help many aspiring models get where they want to go more quickly. I was never a professional model and so have only helped her with this book as a journalist with more than a decade of professional experience. When it was done, though, I wondered if maybe I, too, could succeed at modeling! (Just kidding, Deb.)

We hope you get all the answers you need in these pages or find resources here that will provide you with those answers. The next time we open a glamour magazine, we hope to see your picture smiling back at us, helping to bring a little more beauty into the world.

—Skip Press

Introduction

"*S*hoot for the moon, and even if you miss, you'll land among the stars." That was the quote that fell out of my coworker's fortune cookie.

"Here, you take it. You need it more than I do," my friend said as he handed me the tiny piece of paper. I taped it on the first page of my new day planner and finished writing out a list of all the agencies I planned to visit during my first week in New York. That quote stayed with me throughout my journey.

I'm proud of this book for many reasons. This is the first book my husband, Skip, and I have written together, and it has allowed me the opportunity to share my knowledge of the modeling business. I hope that by reading this book, you will decide what direction you want to take and avoid some of the pitfalls that throw so many models off course. I hope you will find a way to set your sights on what you want and make your dreams come true. I share my experiences throughout this book, so

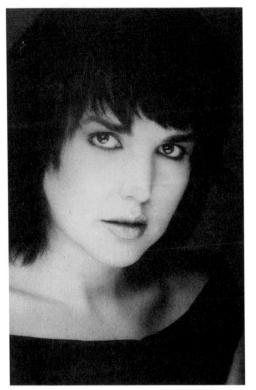

Debbie Press. Photographer Jeff Flax. Makeup Jane Arnold.

when you come to segments written in the first person, know that these are real events from my own modeling career.

My modeling journey began with a glance through the local Sunday newspaper in my hometown of Beckley, West Virginia. For some reason, my eyes locked on a small ad that read:

Modeling Contest. Under Size 12 Need Not Apply. Big Beauties and Little Women of New York needs new faces in their full-figure division. Twelve finalists will be selected and flown to New York City to compete for cash, prizes and modeling contracts.

"I could do that," I thought to myself. After all, I had the required full figure. Other people would tell me, however, that it was a silly idea. At age twenty–three, I still lived in a small town in southern West Virginia where I grew up. I had a fine job with a local coal company. For some reason, though, I could not get that little ad out of my mind.

Why? Because until I saw it, I never knew there were modeling opportunities for large–sized women.

For the first time since high school, I started to take care of myself. For a variety of reasons, my self-esteem had plummeted after graduation. My mother had been ill with cancer, and after a long battle she died when I was in my first year of college. I became depressed, which caused me to gain a lot of weight and drop out of college. But after seeing that small ad in the newspaper about "large-sized" models, I became inspired. For once, there was a possibility of an exciting new future–and excitement was something that had been missing in my life for quite some time.

I invested in a new hairstyle, started to learn about makeup, and gradually changed my overall appearance. My wardrobe went from black and dull to bright and exciting. When I discovered that most popular full-figure models wore a size 12 or 14, I lost weight. After a few months of exercise, eating right, and a more positive mental attitude, I started to feel great about myself. It wasn't long before friends and family began to notice and comment on the change.

I finally made it to a size 16. In order to compete in the Big Beauties contest, I needed two photos. I found John Blankenship, a photographer, who soon became one of my most inspiring and supportive friends. He immediately became enthused about the contest, and about my dream to go to New York and model. John shot several rolls of film to get two suitable shots for the Big Beauties competition. Then John continued to work with me, helping me develop a level of comfort while working in front of a camera.

I decided not to wait around for the Big Beauties contest. I wanted to be a model no matter what the judges decided. The odds against actually "making it" never occurred to me. At age twenty-three, I was planning a career in a profession teeming with sixteen-year-old, size-8 girls.

I found a modeling agency in a nearby city and became their first and only plus-size model. Some of the local stores were thrilled to finally have someone to model large-size fashions. The agency was so pleased, they sponsored me in a modeling competition held in Washington, D.C.

The contest, it turned out, was a way for me to meet an agent from Big Beauties without having to go to New York. In order to compete, I had to learn the art of walking the "catwalk." Remember how Scarlett O'Hara floated down the stairs at Twelve Oaks in *Gone With the Wind* as if she didn't have legs under that hoop skirt? Well, that's how models should glide across a runway. No shaking, wiggling, or bouncing.

Easy to describe, hard to do. A model's walk is achieved with lots of sweat, sore muscles, and by tucking a quarter in your tush and holding it there as you walk (that stops the wiggling). Of course, once you learn to tighten up your derriere, you can do away with the quarter. This technique, taught by Martin Snaric, a New York runway king, took months of rehearsal before I perfected it. Our modeling school sponsored a workshop taught by Martin two months prior to the convention. I benefited so much from it, I signed up for a private lesson.

If I could name one thing that helped me more than anything to create an image filled with self-confidence and grace, it would be my good fortune in finding Martin. Andy Warhol called him "the pop star of the runway" with good reason. His fame from teaching the secrets of a beautiful walk has landed him spots on shows like the *Late Show with David Letterman, Entertainment Tonight,* and *Good Morning, America.*

Basic movements can be very significant in the way you present yourself and the level of confidence you're able to project. By the time I walked across the runway for the judges in Washington, D.C., Martin could tell that I had spent three solid months of "walking the walk." He applauded wildly. Afterward, he nodded from across the stage in approval. I knew I had performed well, and the Big Beauties' agent was in the front row. The Big Apple was only one interview away, and I was prepared to meet the "big beauty" herself in a few hours.

As long as I live, I will never forget meeting the agent from Big Beauties & Little Women. She sat in front of me, along with one of her professional models. I was thrilled to meet them and was in awe of the Big Beauties model. Somehow, I managed to hand them my portfolio without shaking. I felt a wave of shock, though, as they started to snicker and laugh at my photographs. I had worked so hard to put my book together. As the agent closed the cover of my book and handed it back to me, she sneered, "You'll never work in New York!" Those words seemed to carry an echo as I started to hear them over and over again. "You just don't have the look," she added.

I managed to find the elevator and couldn't wait to get up to my room so I could let go of the emotional impact from this meeting. Thank God for Martin Snaric. The runway king managed to squeeze into the elevator with me and asked anxiously, "So, what happened with Big Beauties?" Still frozen, I repeated the harsh words that had just punctured my dream. Martin looked straight in my eyes and said with total conviction,

"Prove her wrong!" The moment was a turning point for me. His statement filled my heart and soul with a burning desire to succeed and remained with me throughout my career as a model. It was then that I knew I would find a way to make my modeling dream come true.

Later that evening, I again had to face the vice president of Big Beauties. As it turned out, she was one of the agents selected to pass out trophies and congratulate the winners from the competitions. It was an absolute pleasure to shake Miss "Big Beauties'" hand and receive my first-place trophy in runway presentation. Our eyes locked for a moment, and I smiled, quietly saying to myself, "Yes, I *will* work in New York!"

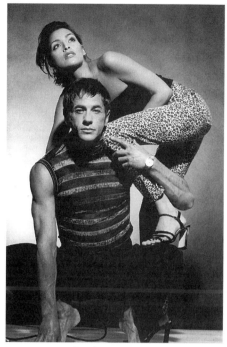

Martin Snaric with Lesley Wayne. Photo by Claus Eggers. © 1999 Claus Eggers.

With one great big dream, the support of a wonderful family, and a small bit of savings, I quit my job and moved to New York City. As I walked to the small plane at our tiny local airport, waving good-bye to my family was one of the hardest things I had ever done. But I had made my decision.

Six months after arriving in the city, I signed a two-year modeling contract with one of the biggest and best agencies in the business—the legendary Ford Modeling Agency. The next three years were spent going on "testings" and "go-sees," working with professional photographers, pounding the pavement, interviewing with clients, walking the runway, working as a fit model, doing catalog work, and modeling jewelry and fur coats. Sometimes I had six "go-sees" stretched out all over Manhattan. I fought people traffic, ducked in doorways to change shoes, and carried half a beauty shop in my shoulder bag. Sometimes they would say, "We love you," and sometimes they would bark, "Next!"–and there were always about fifty other models waiting along with me, competing for that one job.

Oddly enough, after I moved to New York, I found that I kept losing weight. When I started modeling for Ford, I wore a size 14. Within a few months, I dropped to a size 12. The agency kept telling me, "Don't lose another pound, or we can't use you." I had to eat pizza and ice cream just to maintain a size 12 and continue modeling in the plus-size category. Finally, it was no use. I hit a size 10 and immediately found that I was out of the large-size market. There were fewer "go-sees" and jobs in the "Today's Woman" division.

New York was filled with opportunities, and it was time for me to move on and discover what I wanted to pursue next. Of course, that's about the time I met Skip. Not long after we first said hello in the lobby of a small theater, I was ready to take another chance. Six months later, I moved to southern California and married my writer beau.

I've never regretted "shooting for the moon" and pursuing my dreams. Modeling was a stepping-stone to opportunities I would have never known had I not taken the chance. When I first began researching this book, my first thoughts were about what modeling did for me and what I wanted to share with others.

Modeling filled me with self-confidence and poise. I learned how to deal with rejection and cold, harsh words. I experienced how having a burning desire to achieve something can drive you straight to success, no matter what anyone tells you to the contrary. I learned the art of remaining focused on a goal. I learned that you really can get what you want if you truly put your mind to it. And I found out that you should never let anyone get away with telling you that you can't do it, when you believe in your heart that you can. I didn't become famous, nor did I earn a tremendous amount of money. Although I only modeled for three years, it brought me to bigger and better things, like meeting my husband. And because of all these things, I would recommend modeling to anyone.

—Debbie Press
debbiepress@yahoo.com

CHAPTER ONE

The World of Modeling

*"Far away there in the sunshine are my highest aspirations. I may not
reach them, but I can look up and see their beauty, believe in them and
try to follow where they lead."*

LOUISA MAY ALCOTT

*I*t is easy to understand why a mod-
eling career sounds appealing. Glamorous clothing, constant attention
from makeup and hair professionals, and seeing themselves in print is a
fantasy for women around the world. Walking down a runway in a designer gown to the beat of hip music, with cameras flashing all around, is
thrilling to even think about, much less experience. Or how about traveling all around the world, all expenses paid, to shoot in exotic locations?
A lot of models begin their careers in places like Paris or Milan. And then,
of course, there's the money, which can be extraordinary. Today, models
who achieve a high level of success earn more money in a week than
most people earn in a year. Here is what some of the most well-known
models earn yearly, according to *Business Age* (August 14, 1998):

Elle MacPherson .... $40.3 million   Cindy Crawford .... $37.7 million

Claudia Schiffer .... $36.0 million   Naomi Campbell .... $28.9 million

Kate Moss .... $26.3 million

Christy Turlington .... $23.7 million

Helena Christensen ..... $15.8 million

Tyra Banks .... $8.8 million

Laetitia Casta .... $5.3 million

Stephanie Seymour ... $24.6 million

Karen Mulder .... $19.3 million

Eva Herzigova .... $12.3 million

Niki Taylor .... $6.1 million

Given those figures, it's easy to agree with *Webster's Dictionary*, which defines the word "model" as "a person worthy of imitation." In the early 1930s, John Robert Powers opened the first modeling agency in New York. By the end of that decade, the average model earned $5 an hour. That is less than minimum wage today, but back then it was a fortune. Modeling wages really took off when Elite Model Management opened its doors in 1977. John Casablanca's agency portrayed its models as sexier than the girl next door, and the sleek marketing of its models quickly put Elite's girls in a celebrity category, boosting rates for all models.

The aforementioned models are the cream of the crop, the rare few who achieve superstardom. But what about the thousands of nameless models who grace the pages of catalogs and print ads? Although you probably couldn't name a handful of them, they have very successful and lucrative careers. They enjoy steady six-figure incomes and travel all over the world, often with their expenses paid. In contrast, many hopeful models become affiliated with an agency only to discover they don't get enough bookings to support themselves.

Depending on the city where you are based, the average income from modeling ranges from $150 to $1,500 a day, depending on variables such as location, type of work, your experience, and type of client. You'll likely start out slow. Sometimes a model's week is filled with "go-sees" and "testings"; you might only have one booking for $150. That's not much money to live on for one week. Even some of the supermodels will tell you that it was rough getting started. In a *Los Angeles Times Magazine* cover story dated September 21, 1997, superstar model Elle MacPherson recalled how difficult and expensive it was in the beginning, what with all the clothes to buy, rent to pay, and the cost of getting around New York. "I didn't earn any money for years," she said. "I lived on trail mix."

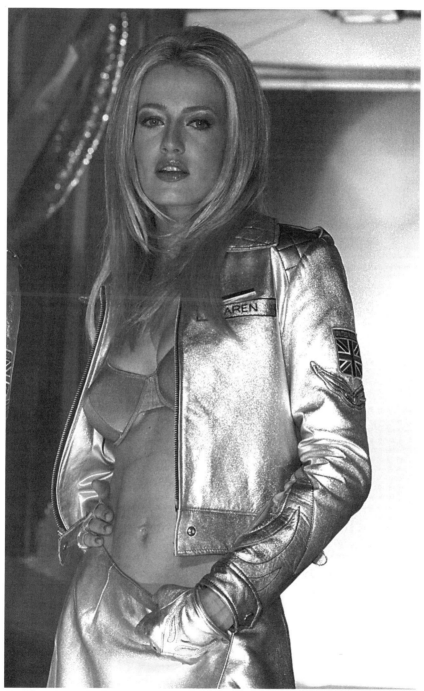

Photo by Andrew Richard. © Canvas 42, Inc.

Where You Need to Live

Although there are modeling schools and agencies in most average-size towns across the United States, if you want a career as a model, your chances of success are greater if you live in a major city. The largest, highest-paying markets in the United States are New York, Miami, Chicago, Dallas, and Los Angeles. There is also a significant amount of work to be found in Boston, Houston, Phoenix, San Francisco, and Washington, D.C. However, New York is the heartbeat of the fashion industry. Many of the major, well-known agencies based in New York also have agencies in other cities. Elite, for example, has offices in Miami, Chicago, and Los Angeles.

In New York, a model can find editorial, catalog, advertising, and runway work. And you don't have to be a superstar to earn a decent living. But what about other cities? The good news is, you do not need to go to New York to have a successful career as a model. There are major markets in other parts of the country where a model can build a successful and rewarding career. Boston, Dallas, Houston, Miami, Phoenix, San Francisco, and Washington, D.C., offer catalog work, and you can find editorial, TV, and catalog work in Los Angeles.

Modeling opportunities are available in most cities in the United States. Work is available in local retail stores, advertisements, and fashion shows, but if you want to consider modeling as a profession, you must examine the major markets in the United States and learn what opportunities exist in those areas. Above all, you must be willing to travel.

It All Begins at Home

The advantage of starting out locally is not only the experience you gain, but the opportunity to see if you like the work. Many young models think working in front of a camera will be fun, but when actually doing a shoot, they discover they don't like it. Many young people discover, after they get a taste of modeling, that they have more talent or interest in another area, like photography or makeup artistry.

The Ever-Changing Business

The modeling industry is always active. If you are a student, you might want to start in the summer. American designers present their spring collections usually around October or November and their fall collections in March or April. You need to learn things like this and keep abreast of the latest likes and dislikes. Part of your job as an aspiring model is to keep on top of what's going on in the fashion world. In this business, trends come and go so quickly one could easily compare it to the day-to-day changes in computer technology.

One recent, pleasing trend in fashion is the portrayal of more "realistic" women. The popularity of the new magazine *Mode* is partially due to the fact that the average American woman weighs around 145 pounds and wears between a size 12 and 14. It's about time we saw a substantial shift in those emaciated visual images we've seen in fashion magazines, advertisements, and catalogs over the past few decades. According to *Chemical & Engineering News*, a study comparing fashion models to "normal" women and women with eating disorders found that the models were significantly underweight on the basis of body-mass index but heavier than anorexic women. One has to wonder if the psychological health of women would improve if more realistic images were prominent in American culture. A psychological study in 1995 found that three minutes spent looking at models in a fashion magazine caused 70 percent of women to feel depressed, guilty, and shameful. Perhaps that's why "plus-size" modeling has taken off in recent years. We now have a role model, Emme, who at a size 14 to 16, has achieved great fame as a "plus-size" model. (Like only the very top celebrities, she is known by a single name.) She landed a Revlon cosmetics contract and is hosting E! Channel's *Fashion Emergency*.

The early nineties saw trends like "grunge" and "heroin chic." Thankfully, this has evolved into a healthier, "girl-next-door" look. Some considered 1999 to be the "year of the dimple." After years of sad and serious-faced models, the smile returned. Smiling these smiles were more African-American, Hispanic, and Asian models in editorial, advertising, and catalog print, as well as on the runway. Such trends speak well of the future of the modeling business.

Another trend that is good news for those models that don't consider themselves to be supermodel material is the recent popularity among advertisers for models with more average looks. According to an April 10, 1997, article in *Los Angeles Times Magazine*, Monique Pillard, president of Elite Model Management, indicated, "Models now are girls the person in the street can relate to. They aren't as perfect as the supermodels were. It's a new look that's popular now, and they even walk differently."

The demise of the supermodel is greatly discussed by industry professionals. Many will not even say the word "supermodel" because the term has become so outdated and controversial. Most fashion business pros believe that, since supermodels commanded too much money, clients began using less-known models at a much-reduced rate out of pure economic survival. For example, some of the supermodels were earning between $15,000 and $20,000 per fashion show and refused to cut their fees. Others report that industry professionals got tired of the spoiled attitude, which was highlighted by Linda Evangelista's famous comment, "We won't get out of bed for less than $10,000." In an *Us* article by Ariel Levy and Steve Garbarion, Calvin Klein proclaimed that people aren't "interested in models anymore" and promptly canned Kate Moss. "Kate was the last of the supermodels," says Amy Astley, beauty director of Vogue. "The girls who are working now, nobody even knows their name." All of these things explain why top fashion magazines started using movie stars, like Michelle Pfeiffer or Gwyneth Paltrow, and other celebrities, like Oprah Winfrey and Hillary Rodham Clinton, for their covers. In fact, major agencies now have a list of actresses they represent for print work.

Although some believe supermodels have seen their day, others believe they'll never die and that there will always be those few who achieve great fame and fortune as models. Maybe one of them will be you.

Do You Have "The Look"?

Tall, lanky models have been the ideal for decades, and it is no different today. Thin and 5'9" is the look most agents are interested in. Fortunately, there is more flexibility now than there was in the past. Most agencies will tell you that they will consider shorter models, and there's certainly room for petites and plus–size models in the business, as well as character models, athletic models, and older models.

If you really want to be a model but think you don't stand a chance because you have some flaw or imperfection, you could be wrong. Aimee Mullins was born without fibulae, which are the outer bones between the ankles and knees. Her legs were amputated from the knees down when she was one year old. Because of the use of prosthetics, however, she has played softball, run races, and modeled for magazines and on the runway in Europe. According to *Cosmopolitan's* April 1999 issue, Aimee moved to Manhattan "to pursue modeling and acting while promoting H.O.P.E. (Helping Others to Perform with Excellence), a nonprofit organization that raises funds for people in need of prosthetics."

Even if you sign a contract with an agent, you should be prepared to pay the bills via other means until your modeling can support you. One cannot emphasize enough the importance of having a back–up plan, like a second career goal in mind when you begin your pursuit of this profession. Modeling is something that most do for only a short period of time before moving on to some other career, educational pursuit, or business.

Your Future in Modeling

How much of an impact will high technology have on the fashion industry? Most industry professionals refuse to believe models will ever be replaced by computer creations, but digital imagery has certainly come a long way in enhancing and changing the images used in fashion photography.

Although it is hard to conceive a day when portfolio books will be secondary to images transmitted and viewed on a computer, that day could soon arrive. When technology allows images to be viewed relatively instantly via cable and DSL modems, as opposed to the time it currently takes to download them at 56K speeds, computer viewing may become the preferred method, or at least gain equal footing.

The use of the Internet makes sense in the fashion industry–images of models can be viewed in seconds from anywhere in the world, and so more agencies are putting up Web sites each day. This technology allows agencies outside of the major markets to compete internationally as well as acquire models and market them worldwide.

Modeling is one of the most difficult fields to break into. It can be a wonderful opportunity to earn a lot of money, travel internationally, experience other cultures, and have a lot of fun. On the downside, it can be lonely, brutal, and eat away at your self-esteem. It is not a profession for a weak, immature individual. If you are strong, thick-skinned, determined, mature, and have a solid emotional foundation, you can reap the benefits and enjoy a lucrative modeling career. And just maybe, millions of people around the world will know your face, if not your name.

CHAPTER TWO

The Different Types of Modeling

"Let the world know you as you are, not as you think you should be,
because sooner or later, if you are posing, you will forget the pose,
and then where are you?"

FANNIE BRICE, AMERICAN COMEDIENNE AND SINGER

*I*f you've ever thought about being
a model, you have probably imagined yourself appearing on the cover of
Vogue or posing in a gorgeous gown in the center section of a top magazine. Or perhaps you have seen yourself walking down the runway in an
exotic designer ensemble with paparazzi flashing all around. These types
of modeling are certainly the most glamorous and well known, but there
are many other types of opportunities to consider.

You might be surprised to learn that some of the other types of modeling actually pay more money. In fact, doing a cover for a magazine or
being chosen for an "editorial" shoot (the top of the line, the next best
thing to a cover) pays significantly less than modeling for a commercial
ad or catalog. Models may earn only $150 for the entire day for shooting
a magazine cover, compared to $150–$300 per hour for catalog work.
Being on the cover of a magazine or featured in an editorial, however, is
not only prestigious, it can help launch a model's career. Once the model

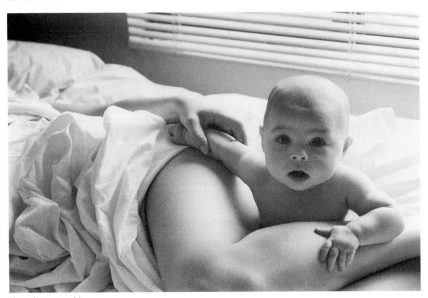

Photo by Erin Ashley.

appears on the cover of a magazine or does an editorial, the tear sheets are put into her book and/or used on her composite card. Quite often, the model's career takes off from there, as she subsequently lands everything from advertising campaigns to work with top designers in fashion shows.

If you're not the right type to succeed as a high-fashion model, you can pursue a very lucrative career by finding the type of modeling that's right for you. Not everyone can become a cover girl or *Vogue*'s next fashion darling. So what if catalog or advertising work isn't as glamorous as fashion editorials or magazine covers? The opportunities are more plentiful, and models of all types are used for print work.

Print Work

"Print work" refers to the printed photographs used in magazines, catalogs, product packaging, greeting cards, billboards, brochures, or any other type of printed material used to advertise a product. There are many different types of print work that use of a wide variety of models.

High-Fashion Modeling

When you see the fashion layouts in *Vogue* or any of the other major fashion magazines, you are looking at high-fashion models. These same models appear in classic fashion advertisements, like those that advertise a designer's collection.

High-fashion models generally share certain characteristics: They are long, lean, and have unique or exotic features. Although these models can vary in age, height, weight, and size, most are between the age of thirteen and twenty-five, are 5'8" to 5'11" in height, and wear a size 6 or 8. But as in other types of modeling, there are certainly exceptions. For example, Kate Moss is considered a high-fashion model, yet her height has been reported in numerous articles as only 5'7". Her career took off when Calvin Klein chose her to do his advertisements and runway shows.

Editorial Print Work

Most models consider editorial print work to be the most interesting and desirable of print media, perhaps because it's the most creative. An editorial model must be able to take direction and be very flexible in working with the professionals on the set. In editorial work, the model will help create the mood of the shoot. Most of the time, the model will put a lot more energy into an editorial shoot than she would for a catalog job. For instance, you might have to jump in the air, stretch your body across some strange object and hold the pose, or do something bizarre like float on water in a designer gown.

Editorials are created by magazine editors and staffers who hand pick every visible thing: the theme, fashions, location, props, and models. Editorials are not designed to sell a product; they tell a fashion story. The story refers to the series of photographs that are set against the same color backdrop or are taken at a specific location. Fashion stories carry out a theme. Most of the time, only a few models are used in a fashion story, and sometimes only one model is featured.

Many models begin their careers abroad because many fashion magazines are produced in Europe. Some of the major markets there include Milan, Paris, Madrid, London, and Munich. Sydney, Australia, is also a

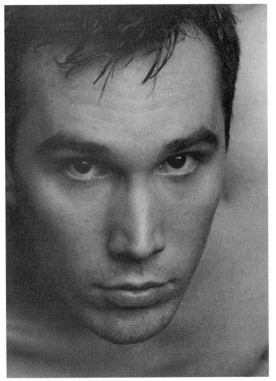

Photo by Stephen Clark. PBSC New York. © 1999 Stephen Clark.
Model: Brian. Makeup: Angela Gallagher.

major international market. Fashion magazines in these cities are quite different than what you'll find in the United States.

Top professionals in the fashion industry claim Italian *Vogue* is the top fashion magazine in the world. If at all possible, try to get copies of Italian *Vogue* and other foreign fashion magazines. Although foreign magazines are more expensive than their American counterparts, viewing them will give you an idea as to what is involved with editorial work on the international scene. There's quite a difference between international fashion print and that of the United States. You'll see some of the most interesting, artistic, and bizarre fashion photography imaginable in foreign magazines.

Commercial Print

Commercial print models are those who primarily work for catalogs and advertisements. Although the height and size requirements are generally the same as for high fashion, most commercial print models tend to have a look with which the consumer can relate. This not only refers to the "all-American, girl-next-door" look, but to a wide variety of types.

Catalog

As mentioned earlier, catalog work usually pays substantially more than editorials. This type of work features the display of merchandise, which includes everything from fashion to food. In addition to major department-store catalogs, like Spiegel or JC Penney, there are many mail-order catalog companies in existence. There are even catalogs that sell subscriptions to catalogs. And they all use models.

One of the best things about catalog modeling, aside from the money you earn, is the fact that physical requirements vary widely. There are hundreds of specialty catalogs on the market today that cater to specific types—from women who wear size 12 and up to mature models who are in their forties or fifties. There are catalogs that specialize in shoes, wigs, bathing suits, hats, jewelry, lingerie—you name it. And all of them use a variety of models to sell their wares.

In terms of fashion, a number of mail-order catalogs have a high-quality, artistic look. *Victoria's Secret* is a great example. These companies invest a lot of money for a well-designed catalog. They hire top photographers and models, and the print work often resembles the look of editorials.

The emphasis in modeling for a catalog is on the clothing, not the model; the purpose is to show the clothing or merchandise in the best possible way. Generally, a model is directed to move slowly and purposefully in catalog work. Most movements are fairly standard, so as the model begins to work in this category, the posing becomes very natural and second nature.

Catalog Posing and Pay

When I first moved to New York, I watched a catalog shoot from my window and was amazed at how little the model actually moved. She was dressed in a business suit and looked as if she were walking down the stairs of a brownstone building. For the longest time, she slowly took one single step, over and over again.

To get an idea of how standard catalog posing can be, lay out four to five catalogs from different companies and study the models. You will see very similar poses in each book. This exercise will give you a feel for how to pose for a catalog booking. Practice these poses in front of a full-length mirror, and move to see how the garment looks and feels and what your best angles are.

As previously mentioned, catalog work pays anywhere from $150 to

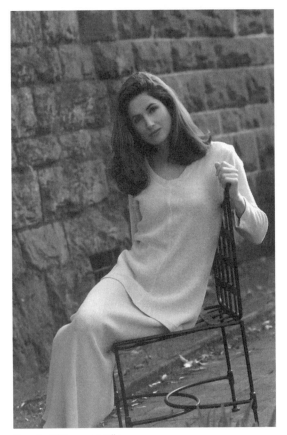

Photo by Bill Lemon. © Bill Lemon.

$300 per hour to $1,200 to $2,500 per day. A catalog booking can take anywhere from a few hours to a full week. Some bookings will be shot in a studio, while others are shot on location.

Most models that work for catalogs on a steady basis find that they are able to enjoy a long and prosperous career. You've probably heard the standard belief that models don't work much past their mid–twenties because that age is considered old in this business. While it can be true that models who work in the high–fashion/editorial end of modeling depend on the whim of current trends, it doesn't have to be that way.

Stephanie Averill, a very successful model who travels extensively and appears in major advertisements and national print, has worked in everything from editorials to catalogs. Her long and prosperous career is a great example of a model who continues to enjoy stability as a model after several years in the business. Stephanie was approached about modeling while visiting in Paris; she ended up staying there and working, but it didn't take her long to discover the downside of the modeling world as she encountered everything from playboys to model groupies. "My college education helped attribute to my success," she says. "I was more mature, was able to say no, and felt as if others took me more seriously and respected me more. My education and the fact that I started out at an older age–older than the fourteen-year-olds–has had a significant impact on my career."

Sometimes models are pushed into early retirement because they refuse to do catalog work when they've been doing editorials and major advertisements. Generally, however, the longevity of a model's career depends on the model's attitude, professionalism, and desire to continue success.

Advertising

This type of work refers to advertisements that appear in magazines, brochures, packaging of products, even billboards. Instead of modeling for a publication, as in editorial work or for a catalog company, you model directly for the company that makes or designs the product. The rates for advertising models are usually higher than catalog work, particularly if an exclusive agreement is negotiated. For instance, if a model signs an exclusive agreement to work for a cosmetics company, say Estée Lauder, she agrees that for a stated amount of time she will only model cosmetics for that particular product line. In other words, you won't see her in a Maybelline ad during that time. The client pays a sum in addition to the model's rates for exclusive rights, which compensates for other opportunities the model will not be able to pursue while under exclusive contract. If you look through a year's worth of women's magazines, you'll notice models like Niki Taylor in the Cover Girl ads, or Elizabeth Hurley modeling for Estée Lauder. You'll see Cindy Crawford modeling for Revlon, and in the same magazine, you'll see her modeling for a designer like Ellen Tracy, or for Omega watches. But you won't see Cindy modeling another cosmetics line. The look of the ads will change, but for a given amount of time, the same model will represent the product, becoming the face of that product—its spokesperson.

The terms of exclusive agreements are confidential, but for major products (like Revlon or Estée Lauder) the amount can blossom to an amount more than six figures. The specifics are negotiated according to various factors, such as the length of time the ad will run, the number of days of usage, or the length of time the model will be committed to represent the product. Although this limits the model's choices in doing similar work for other companies, it gives her a lot of exposure and helps to build her image.

Advertising also utilizes more "real people" models for its ads, depending on the product. A soap ad, for example, might most effectively use an ordinary looking model.

Start studying advertisements and print work in various types of magazines. A great place to sit and browse through magazines is in your local library. Look through all types of magazines, like *Better Homes and Gardens, Woman's Day,* and *Psychology Today,* to see the different types of models used in stories and advertisements. Think about which of these advertisements you can see yourself doing. This will help you to pinpoint the type of print work that suits you best. Study the different images of models and think about the pose, expression, and general mood of each print.

Parts or Specialty Work

Specialty models are those who have perfect features, such as hands, feet, legs, teeth, face, or incredible hair. Petite models are good candidates for this type of work because of their delicate features; specifically, small hands and feet. Most female hand models wear a ring size of 4 to 7, and female shoe models wear a size 5 or 6.

Advertisements that feature parts models represent products such as hand lotion, panty hose, shoes, lipstick, and many others. Parts models are also frequently used for television commercials and command a higher rate.

In order to model in this category, you have to maintain perfect features. For instance, hands and feet must be extremely well manicured, with no protruding veins, marks, nicks, or cuts. A parts model must avoid activities that could affect the quality of the specific body part(s). Professional models that make the commitment to specialize as a parts model can often enjoy a longer career, but it takes a dedicated individual. For instance, Laura Gens of Parts Models in New York has enjoyed her career as a parts model for nearly ten years. In fact, most of us have probably seen Laura's hands, legs, feet, eyes, or lips in advertisements. Laura commented that one of the most difficult things about being a parts model is that you have to be so careful about everything. "You can't do normal activities, like bike riding, mountain climbing, washing dishes, cleaning.

You're very limited in what you can do."

Although clients hire professionals to do manicures and pedicures on shoots, as a parts model, you have to keep your hands and feet well maintained. Laura has a strict regimen she follows each day. She takes calcium and other supplements that are good for the nails and skin. She constantly moisturizes, using combinations of baby ointment and Vaseline. At night she uses a lot of moisturizing products and sleeps with white beauty gloves, a sweat suit, and white cotton socks. It sounds like a lot of work, but for Laura it has become routine. "This lifestyle forces good grooming habits– you find what works for you and just do it."

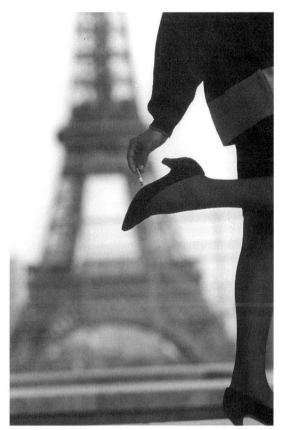

Photo by Karim Ramzi. © Karim Ramzi.

Ellen Sirot is a hand model with Parts Models who has also enjoyed a long career. She trained as a dancer, which she believes enhanced her career as a hand model. This is easy to understand when you think of the gracefulness of a ballerina. Her advice to those who want to break into this type of modeling is to have professional photographs taken and send them to an agent who represents parts models. Just be sure you're up for the challenge. As Ellen states: "It's a twenty–four–hour–a–day, seven–day–a–week commitment. You have to be willing to take care of yourself and know that you will be giving up a lot of normal activities. You even have to avoid activities that will build up muscles in your hands." Just like other types of modeling, parts is also very competitive. You have to

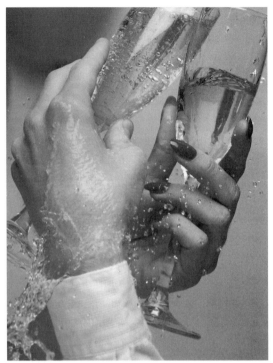

Photo by Karim Ramzi. © Karim Ramzi.

be committed, professional, and do a good job. Sometimes you work long hours and have to hold uncomfortable positions for a long period of time.

If you think that you have perfect body parts and want to pursue this type of modeling, you should have professional photographs taken of your specific parts and send them to agencies that offer this specialty division. Unlike other types of modeling, if you want to be considered seriously, you will have to supply agents with professional photographs instead of snapshots. Be sure to include all of your statistics on the photograph: shoe size, ring size, and glove size, along with your name, address, and telephone number.

Glamour Modeling

You might think glamour modeling includes elegant gowns, diamonds or pearls, with the model's hair twisted into an elegant do. If so, you might be surprised to learn that this type of modeling often refers to partial or full nudity.

A few years ago, posing nude was not acceptable if you wanted to pursue a serious modeling career. But today, models are posing nude in legitimate mainstream magazines, and usually more than one nude or seminude advertisement or fashion layout can be found in most magazines. Even top models have posed nude for editorial work and advertisements, and some have appeared topless on the runway. For instance, according to a December 1, 1998, article in *The Village Voice*, Bruce Weber shot a nude Kate Moss for a fashion magazine called *Joe's*, in which Kate rolls on the grass and blows bubbles with two naked children.

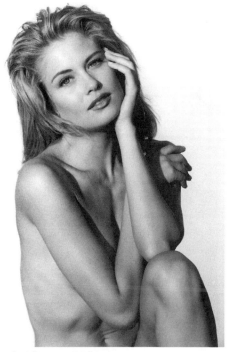

Photo by Bill Lemon. © Bill Lemon.

In the world of fashion and advertising, nude shots that are tasteful, artistic, and beautifully photographed are perfectly acceptable. Famous photographers, like Herb Ritts, Arthur Elgort, or Bruce Weber, shoot most of the prints. Posing nude for fashion magazines or advertisements no longer carries the stigma it did a few years ago. Of course, there are sleazy publications that are filled with nudes, but those have nothing to do with building a career as a fashion model. Posing nude is not something a model should feel she must do to get her career off the ground–it's a personal choice. According to *The Wilhelmina Guide to Modeling* by Natasha Esch, some models, like Claudia Schiffer, claim that under no circumstances will they ever pose nude.

Most models are thin, fit, and work very hard to maintain their bodies. Of course, some models hit the gene–pool jackpot and are born with amazing physical attributes that they don't have to struggle to maintain. The majority are proud of their bodies and are not bothered by showing off their greatest assets, so it's easy to understand why some models are completely at ease with nudity issues. Lingerie and swimwear models fit in this category. There are also many models from other cultures who find nudity, or posing topless, more acceptable.

The bottom line is that you must decide for yourself what your own boundaries will be when it comes to nudity. You should never be pres-

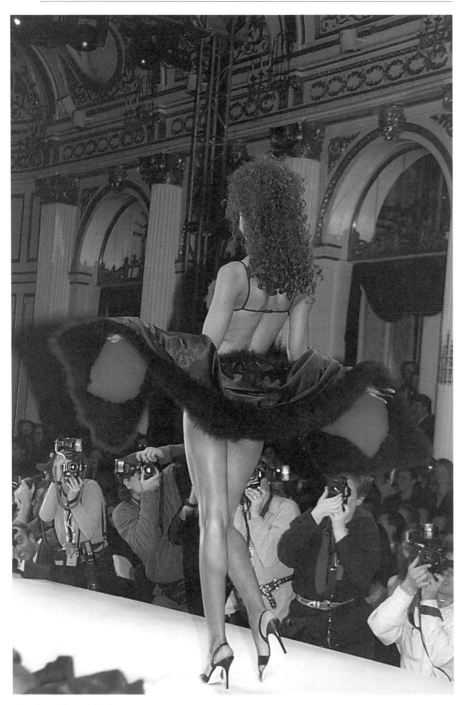

Photo by Andrew Richard. © Canvas 42, Inc.

sured by anyone to pose nude, nor should you feel bad about yourself if you decide to keep your clothes on. Karim Ramiz, a successful fashion photographer in Paris, said, "All models, even high fashion models, are eventually asked if they will pose in the nude. So you should solve that problem in advance and decide for yourself what you will and will not do. In Europe, nudity is considered normal and pays extremely well, but in America the rules are still different."

Remember, there are plenty of well-known models that have not posed nude and adamantly claim they never will. Taking your clothes off is not necessarily the fast track to the top.

Runway

This type of modeling is, by far, the most well-known type of live modeling. Although you'll find fashion shows in just about any city across the United States, you will have to work in New York, Paris, or Milan to earn a high salary from runway work. Beginning runway models can earn $250 per hour, while famous models usually command anywhere from $10,000 to $20,000 (or more) per show. Major runway shows take place in the fall (usually September), when designers show off their spring collections, and in the spring (usually March), when the fall collections are shown. These events show off the designer's fashion collections and have become quite extravagant productions.

Designers hire models through modeling agencies to show their new lines. Department stores may hire models for shows, depending on location. Fashion shows are also coordinated through charity organizations.

Victoria's Secret took a different approach to producing its fashion show of 1999. According to Rebecca Quick's February 4th *Wall Street Journal* article, during the Super Bowl, a thirty-second commercial promoted the Victoria's Secret live fashion show on the Web. Within an hour, more than a million viewers visited the Web site to view it on their personal computers. If you haven't had a chance to see the rerun on cable Channel E, you can always log onto *www.victoriassecret.com* and take a look.

Runway models are 5'9" to 6'0" in height and wear a size 8, but there have been exceptions to these requirements. A new model should jump at the chance to work a fashion show for the exposure alone. It's a great way to be seen by designers, photographers, agents, clients, editors of magazines–basically, the top-level professionals of the business. If you're lucky enough to be booked for a fashion show, you will probably get other bookings as a result.

There's a little more to a runway performance than just walking straight down the stage, turning around, and walking back. If you've ever watched a professional fashion show, hopefully you've noticed a precise technique in the way a model walks, turns, or removes a jacket. You should be aware that the "walk" is going to vary, depending on the season, the environment, the designs, and the mood of the set.

$\sim$

Tips for Walking the Walk

One of the easiest ways for the aspiring model to stay on top of the latest techniques in walking the runway is to try to catch fashion shows on cable Channel E. Pay attention to how the models walk, turn, and show the clothing. One standard you'll find in runway technique is the way a model walks with one foot directly in front of the other, as if she's walking on a straight line. Note the way she turns, when she turns, and where she puts her hands.

If you are interested in learning more about runway technique and don't have access to a runway trainer, I recommend investing in a couple of videos. *How to Be a Successful Runway Model* by Shailah Edmonds offers advice for men and women who want to learn how to walk the runway. A beautiful book entitled *Catwalk: Inside the World of the Supermodels*, by Sandra Morris, will take you inside the lives of some of the top models in the business as well as introduce you to the collections, fashion photographers, designers, and magazines.

Martin Snaric, also known as "prince of the runway," offers a few suggestions to improve your posture and stamina—which are not only key for a great runway model, but will also help you appear taller, thinner, more energetic, and self-assured:

• Imagine that you are squeezing a quarter between your buttocks.

By firming up, you won't bounce, and you will support your back, tighten your abs, and straighten your spine.

- Use your lower body muscles for a smoother stride.
- Imagine you are a puppet and a string is pulling you up from the crown of your head, which will elongate the neck and spine.

Snaric has inspired many models, actors, and other professionals to be all that they can be. He says, "Give yourself permission to enjoy and not be ashamed of your incredible desire to be a star. Be proud of all your preparation. With our desire and preparation, we will definitely see opportunities coming out of the universe because of all the work we have done to realize our dreams."

One of the most important things to remember about runway modeling is, if you make a mistake, keep going as if nothing happened. Everyone makes mistakes, even top runway models. Most of the time, you'd never know it. Some models actually incorporate their mistakes into their runway presentation, adding humor so the audience believes they planned it that way.

Be sure to maintain a high level of professionalism when working with the staff and crew who work behind the runway. Even if you're wearing the ugliest garment you've ever seen, you should pretend that it's the most beautiful. Never say anything negative about the fashions you wear.

Last but not least, relax and have fun. Feel the beat of the music and the way the clothes feel on your body, and enjoy the feeling of sharing the new designs with your audience.

~

Interview with
Andrew Richard,
Runway Photographer

For most professional models, runway shows are an incredible experience. To give you an idea as to what runway shows are all about, Andrew Richard, a top runway photographer, shared with us the experience and full flavor of a top New York runway fashion show.

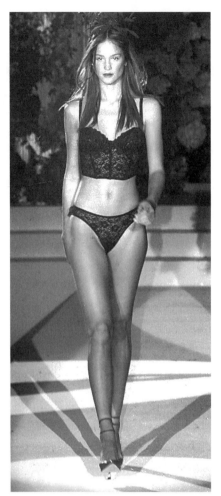

Photo by Andrew Richard. © Canvas 42, Inc.

Press: When did you start shooting fashion shows?

Andrew: Five years ago I began my career on the runways. I discovered a place where I could be free to shoot what I wanted and how I wanted it. The New York runways, for me, are a place where the model can be truly venerated and seen just as she should be. There are no editors or bosses to get on my back and no deadlines to meet. Season after season, newcomers arrive from across the world for their auditions with the top designers. Those lucky enough to be picked will be tomorrow's cover girls. Many turn back home discouraged and never have their dream fulfilled.

Press: Can you describe what a major New York fashion show is like?

Andrew: A two-minute whistle blows loud through the crowd, causing a mad dash for an editor's seat or a dead-center photographer's position. The models, backstage at this moment, begin their adrenaline rush. Some begin to shake from fear, others bite their nails, all try to look cool and calm.

The house lights dim. The designers' music blasts through the giant tents that house the runways as pedestrians in the street walk past outside not knowing the amazing fashion history being written just a few feet away. The crowd becomes motionless. The celebrities, editors, and top buyers in the front row open their designer handouts and, with pen in hand, get ready to circle the designs or models' names that interest them the most.

As the first model steps out, just a foot outside the backstage curtain which gave her security and hid her from the crowd for the last few hours, I, along with a few dozen of the best photographers in the world, begin flashing like a lightning storm.

The model walks closer to me, and, step by step by step, she heads to the front and center spot. Just inches from television cameras, print photographers, and the people who may make her famous for years to come, she stops. For only a moment she is motionless. The camera clicks sound loud to her now. Her dreams are now reality, and all the world is hers.

The energy cannot be described properly in words. The sweat is bursting from every pore in my body. My tie and shirt are soaked in the steam the runway has stirred. And as the music blasts the catwalk, the model turns and walks back slowly to allow us a few more seconds of her beauty. As she reenters backstage she instantly changes gears, from a slow and calculated walk to a frenzied dash to her dressing station. Often she is nude within five seconds. In another minute she will be back

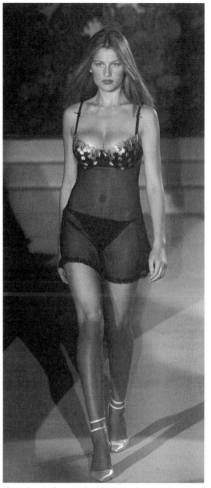

Photo by Andrew Richard. © Canvas 42, Inc.

out to see me again, this time perhaps looking like a completely different person. Perhaps I will notice her. Perhaps *Vogue* will find her look to be the new look of fashion for years to come.

If the model's look is just right, the crowd will roar and applause as loud as a freight train. Backstage, the designer is listening. As her best pieces reemerge backstage, she immediately bags them and marks them for *Vogue* and *Elle* and the top photographers to borrow.

And then, in a second, the music stops. The lights brighten, and before the models can leave the runway the guests begin to run at full speed

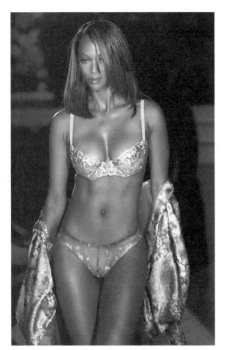

Photo by Andrew Richard. © Canvas 42, Inc.

to the door. They need to hurry and grab a perfect seat at the next show, for in just a few minutes the next designer will be showing six months' worth of hard work to the entire fashion world.

Backstage, the models are hugging and kissing old friends, new ones, and the designer, and wondering, "Did the photographer even notice me?" And yes . . . I notice every thread.

Press: Which shows have been your favorites to shoot and why?

Andrew: Every season a new designer shows up on the scene to surprise and amaze everyone. For the season I just finished up, the award would have to go to Luca Luca for his great collection with sexy, new up-and-coming models. The season before it was Julian McDonald from London, and the season before that it had to be Bob Mackie for his Broadway-style runway show *All That Jazz.*

Press: What kind of schedule do you work during the shows?

Andrew: Scheduling these shows is very difficult. They run every hour on the hour from 9:00 A.M. to 9:00 P.M., Saturday through the following Friday. That's twelve shows a day times seven days straight. At the end of each day I am dropping off film to develop so by the next morning the slides are ready to go out to the magazines and my clients.

Press: What do you like most about shooting the shows?

Andrew: Sipping champagne from a small bottle with a straw.

Andrew Richard is a New York–based fashion photographer and photojournalist. His work can be seen in many publications, both domestic and international. Andrew can be contacted by e-mail at info@canvas42.com or by phone at (516) 791-4191.

~

Fit Modeling

Let's return from the high-profile, fantasy-provoking world of the runway model to other less glamorous, but often lucrative, forms of live modeling. A fit model works as a live mannequin, who can show the movement (and fit) of a garment. Designers use fit models to try on their designs throughout the creative process. Maybe the garment needs a pocket, or some darts for a tighter fit. Maybe the designer wants the skirt to flare out when the model turns around.

The main requirement for this type of modeling is for the model to be a perfect size (usually a size 8), although the size may vary depending on the designer. Full-figures and petites are also utilized for fit modeling.

Often, a fit model has to endure being on her feet for long periods of time as the fabric of a garment is pinned and pulled. Generally, the fit model will try on a stack of garments and work for several hours. The good news is, a fit model usually earns around $150 per hour.

Most fit models also do other types of modeling, since it can be difficult to get enough bookings to work steadily as a fit model and earn a decent living. It is difficult, but certainly not impossible. There are a few models in the business who earn livings as fit models.

Showroom Modeling

As the title indicates, a showroom model works in the designer's showroom and informally models the designer's latest fashions. This type of work is often seasonal, timed around the spring or fall shows. Some designers, however, use models to work in their showrooms on an ongoing basis or when they anticipate a visit by important clients or buyers. In these circumstances, models have the opportunity to practice runway

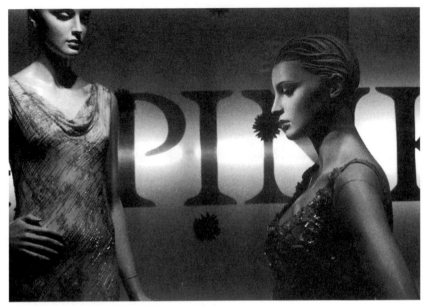

"Pink," New York, 1999. © 1999 Jorgen Hornsten-Gran.

technique, network with industry professionals, and earn steady income.

Jenni Adams, a former showroom girl, sustained her New York modeling career by working in showrooms for fur companies. Jenni is tall and slender, but not "model" thin, which seemed to make her popular with the furriers. "It felt weird at times," she explained. "I had to walk in front of buyers wearing these full-length furs, sometimes with a hat and muff. I mean, who wears a muff in New York? The first audition I had was in a $20,000 chinchilla fur, and the manager told me to walk back and forth in the coat, but do not perspire. I was scared to death, but I guess I didn't let it show, because I got the job."

One of the greatest benefits from becoming a showroom model is the exposure—you never know when it might turn into something bigger and better. For instance, Francesca was noticed in a showroom setting, which led to signing a contract with Wilhelmina. "While in high school I was a junior assistant buyer for a small retail chain based in my hometown of Lawrenceville, New Jersey. I had been asked to accompany the chain's buyer to New York City to visit the various showrooms of the apparel manufacturers. While in one of the showrooms, some of the senior management mistakenly thought I was one of *their* models, which I certainly was not. They said I just had to be a model and so arranged a meeting for me at the Ford agency. I visited Ford, but at that time they were more inclined to sign all-American, blonde-haired, blue-eyed beauties. Well, I'm a dark-haired, brown-eyed girl, so I didn't fit Ford. But they made an appointment for me at Wilhelmina. I visited that same day and was signed on the spot. They changed my name to Kelly Reese, made arrangements for me to room with two other models at the

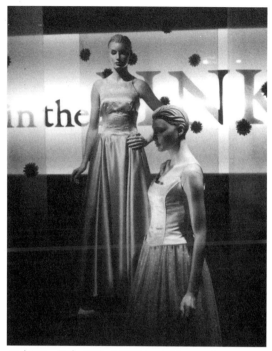

"Pink," New York, 1999. © 1999 Jorgen Hornsten-Gran.

New York Health and Racquet Club, and so began phase one of my modeling career."

Showroom models have to be the perfect size (usually a size 8), although this can vary according to the designer's sample sizes and type of clothing. Large sizes and petites also work as showroom models. The rates are similar, if not a little more, than a fit model, ranging up to $1,000 or more per day.

Promotional Modeling

Often referred to as spokesmodels, promotional models work at sales conventions, trade shows, events, exhibitions, and in stores. They demonstrate products, meet and greet visitors, and distribute literature. Models who work in this category are generally hired to promote products, but many also find themselves handing out awards or giving out samples. There's a variety of work when it comes to promotional modeling.

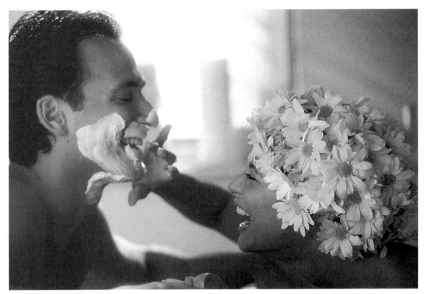

Photo by Gary Jones. Dan Einhorn and Donna DeCianni, Pretty People Model Management, New York, NY. © 1999 Gary S. Jones.

Informal modeling (which at one time was called "tea room" modeling) takes place when a model walks through a store, restaurant, or banquet room modeling various garments. The model usually works two to three hours, models several fashions, and is available to answer questions or give details about the design she is modeling.

If you want to work in this field, you will need to invest in professional photographs and build a composite card. Often an agency chooses models straight from a card without an interview. Although the pay rate is usually not as high as other types of modeling, the bookings can extend over several days. For the entrepreneurial model, it is conceivable to earn a living as a model in this category.

To model in this category, you don't have to be a perfect size 8, 5'8" tall (or more), or under eighteen years of age; you don't even have to be a breathtaking beauty. If you're very people oriented, have a good attitude, enjoy working with the public, and don't mind standing on your feet for long periods of time, this is a type of modeling worth considering. If you've tried to make it as a print model but find that you are not getting enough work to pay the bills, take a look at promotional work.

Television and Film Work

Models are often booked for television commercials, soap operas, videos, industrial films, educational films, or a variety of video and film productions used to advertise products. If you enjoy drama or think you would like to pursue this type of opportunity, find a good acting class. If you live in New York or Los Angeles, there are many types of acting teachers available, and some classes are even geared toward models who want to pursue commercials.

Naturally, you will find a lot of competition when it comes to auditioning for film roles and television commercials. Needless to say, these jobs are very desirable and are sought by actors and actresses, too. If you are in a television commercial, you can earn a lot of money in residuals, and that money can continue to come in for months after the commercial is filmed, depending on how often it is aired. If you do a television commercial and meet specific requirements, you will be able to join the Screen Actors Guild (SAG). Probably the greatest benefit in being able to join SAG is the fact that you can take advantage of a health–care plan and other benefits after you join.

There are a number of resources available if you are interested in breaking into commercials or acting. If you are serious about television commercials and film work, you will find yourself on an entirely different career path than you would take as a model.

CHAPTER THREE

Model Types: Beyond Beautiful

"The future belongs to those who believe in the beauty of their dreams."
ELEANOR ROOSEVELT

*C*ontrary to popular belief, models do not need to be classic beauties with perfect bodies in order to get work. There are venues and markets that provide work for models of all shapes and sizes. In fact, models in specialty categories often enjoy longer careers than high-fashion, editorial types, who are subject to trends and heavier competition.

The key is finding your niche—not only in your own area of specialty, but also in the geographical location most suited to your type. For instance, petite models that find it difficult to work in the major U.S. or European markets often find success in the Asian markets. Many models start out in Japan or Tokyo and work there for a couple of months to gain experience and tear sheets.

There are models who are downright homely who find work. Funny Face in New York or Ugly in London are great examples of agencies that place unusual-looking people. According to Sandra Morris's *The Model*

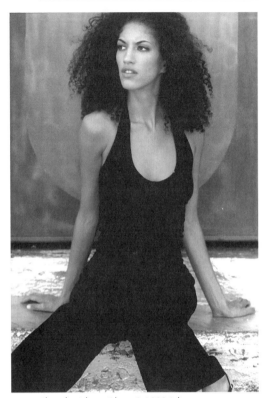

Kimya. Photo by Johnny Olsen. © 1999 Johnny Olsen Photography.

Manual, character models don't have to get on the treadmill of go-sees, nor do they have to spend months working for a pittance while building up a book. Clients will either hire them directly or request them for casting on the strength of their pictures in the agency book. That's not to say that all the models represented by these specialized agencies are "ugly." They represent a wide variety of characters–from beautiful to bizarre.

If you don't fit into the typical tall, thin, fashion-model mold, you might one day consider yourself lucky. As crazy as that may sound, I have known plenty of models that enjoy not being a part of the typical fashion world. For example, in New York, I lived in the same building as a petite Ford model who landed a lot of "extra" roles for soap operas and other television shows. Those opportunities were not extended to conventional tall, thin models. When I modeled in the plus-size division at Ford, I was often the envy of my tall, thin model friends, particularly on Friday nights when we would all go out to dinner, and I was forced to order pizza or pasta because my agency told me I couldn't afford to lose another pound.

Petites

Petite models wear a size 3 to 7 and are between 5'2" and 5'6" in height. Petites are used for catalog work, print ads, editorials for petite-size clothing, and television commercials. Because of petite models' delicate features, they often cross over to parts modeling. For instance, foot or shoe models have small feet, wearing a size 5 or 6 shoe. Petite models can also be booked as beauty models, appearing in ads for facial products or on magazine covers. Designers also book petite models for petite fashion shows or utilize them as fit models.

I once knew a petite model who found it difficult to find steady work in the catalog market. She modeled for a few specialty catalog companies and was able to land a few "extra" parts on soap operas, but she soon found that most of the money she earned came from modeling for romance-novel covers. Even though those bodice-ripping book covers are drawn, they require *live* models. My friend dressed up in camisoles and hoop skirts and typically found herself in a tight, romantic embrace with a male model for hours. To be honest, she wasn't crazy about the work, but it more than paid for her rent while she pursued her modeling career. She was the envy of most of the models who lived in our apartment building who couldn't get a single booking (or a date).

Full-Figure or Large-Size Models

Several years ago, designers became aware of the number of American women who wear a size 12 or larger, and the large-size modeling market emerged. Today, some top agencies, like Wilhelmina and Ford, have large-size divisions. Although a majority of the work for full-figure models is catalog and advertisements, they also appear in editorials for magazines. The international market for large sizes has expanded in Germany, Italy, France, and Sweden. This is still a new and growing field in modeling. As more designers recognize this market as a substantial one, the trend will more than likely grow in editorials. Top fashion magazines, such as *Vogue*, have featured editorials for large-size fashions. A new magazine, *Mode*, was created specifically for this market.

Full-figure models have the same type attributes as standard-size models in that they are tall, well proportioned, and have beautiful, well-structured facial features and clear skin. They are fit and toned, are able to move and stretch freely, and usually wear a size 10 to 20, although the most popular sizes in this market are 12 and 14. Susan Georget of

Wilhelmina says she likes to see models who exhibit clean and natural beauty. Her advice to models who want to establish a long-term career is to "continue to revamp your style and looks. The industry itself continues to look for new talent."

One of the greatest things about being a full-figure model is the fact that one doesn't have to fight to maintain a size 8. Of course, I personally remember struggling to *fill out* a size 12 after becoming a plus-size model. With all the walking and running here and there for go-sees, I kept losing weight. My booker told me that if I wanted to continue to model in this category, I could not lose any more weight. That was a first! As I mentioned previously, I was forced to eat pizza and ice cream, and for the first time in my life, I had trouble keeping the weight on.

A full-figure model approaches her career in the same way a straight-size model does. She goes on testings, puts together her portfolio and a composite card, and goes on as many go-sees as she can. Her rates are equivalent to straight-size models. One of the more important differences is the fact that full-figure models can enjoy a longer career. The age factor is not as strict, although young models are certainly recruited.

Males

Although male models work all over the world, the central place for fashion is in New York. In modeling, males have the same type of opportunities as females. They can find work in magazine editorials, print ads, television commercials, and on the runway. Male models possess a wide range of looks, from youthful to athletic to sophisticated. There's even a market for big and tall men. Most male models are between 5'11" and 6'2" in height, with classic features, high cheekbones, full lips, and well-toned bodies.

Back in the eighties, when the popular age range for male models was twenty to forty years old, men had a potential twenty-year career. According to Franca Palumbo, of Wilhelmina, New York, "If the current trend of utilizing much younger males (teens) continues, a career in high fashion/editorial for males probably won't last more than two years."

But again, these trends change almost as frequently as the wind changes direction.

Of course, some can continue their careers if they are willing to work in smaller markets or catalogs. According to Brian White, a model with Elite L.A., "A steady-working male model can have a much longer than average career than a female model–especially when it comes to commercial work." Since editorial models are often hot for only one season, male models–just like females–should always have their eyes open for other opportunities, whether it is working in a different modeling category or switching gears entirely to a whole new career.

Although this is one of the few professions where women generally make more money than men,

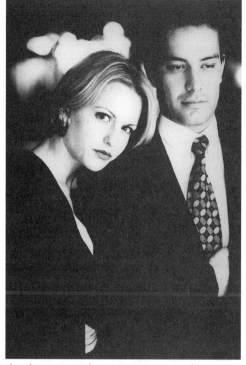

Photo by D. Brian Nelson. © 1999 D. Brian Nelson.

there's some evidence of change, as some of the male models are becoming more well-known and commanding higher rates. Men can earn anywhere from $1,000 to $15,000 per day doing everything from catalog work, covers, advertisements, runway shows, and editorials.

Juniors

Teenage models can be found in magazines like *Sassy, Teen,* and *Seventeen.* It is possible for a large agency to have a thirteen–year–old girl who works in the teenage market, and a more mature–looking thirteen–year–old girl from the same agency booked through the women's division. Often teen models are those who have grown from the children's division or work part–time while going to school. Teens also work in print ads, catalogs, television commercials, and on the runway.

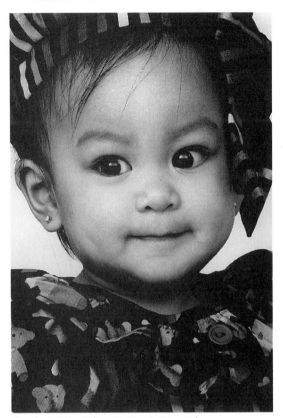

Photo by D. Brian Nelson. © 1999 D. Brian Nelson.

Children

Child models—including babies—can work in catalogs, print ads, television commercials, and sometimes fashion shows. Children need to be very well behaved, outgoing, and flexible to succeed as models. They should be able to take simple directions and not be afraid to try new things.

A successful child model is not always the beautiful, perfect-looking kid. It's often the ordinary, fun-filled kid with freckles or the one who wears glasses who gets the job. Although most parents believe their child is the most beautiful kid on the block, fashion trends make certain types marketable, and those trends come and go. Just because your child isn't right today, it doesn't mean he or she won't be marketable six months from now.

Wendy Rose, an agent in the Children's Division at Ford, looks for kids who are natural, have a fresh face, and have a sparkle in their eye. "When it comes to child models," she explains, "all types are needed." Interestingly enough, Wendy has also seen some kids really blossom as a result of their modeling experience. Unfortunately, child models face rejection, too, just like adult models, so parents need to give their child a solid foundation, help them learn to put rejection aside, and move along to the next opportunity.

There are plenty of reputable agencies that represent children, but beware of agents who ask for a lot of money up front. (See chapter 10,

Avoiding the Dark Side of the Business, which goes into more detail about such rip-offs.) If an agency wants to represent your child, there will more than likely be minimal costs for portfolio and composite photographs. Unfortunately, when it comes to children, there are plenty of disreputable agencies that take advantage of parents who want their kids to enjoy this fun and lucrative opportunity. One of the best sources for finding a good agent for your child is through parents of children who work in the business.

For more information concerning modeling careers for children, see chapter 16.

Mature Models

When most of us think of a mature model, we think of the beautiful, classic-looking, high-fashion model Carmen Dell'Orefice. There are plenty of magazines and catalogs that cater to older adults, and the pages of those publications are filled with mature models.

But Carmen Dell'Orefice has been modeling for a long time. Can you start out as an older model? Absolutely! As long as there are agencies that represent older adults, there will be a demand for mature models.

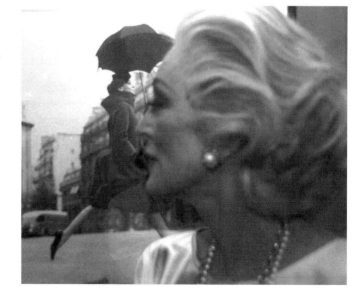

Photo by Andrew Richard.
© Canvas 42, Inc.

The requirements are very similar to that of regular-type models, particularly if you are interested in modeling fashion. But you do have to be realistic and know that there are certain things that will be different for you than for a sixteen-year-old model walking through an agency door. For example, when it comes to testing, it may not be as easy to find photographers to work with. I interviewed an older model named Karen, who said, "It takes a lot of work and effort for an older model. Not everyone wants to work with a 'mature' model."

A mature model should have beautiful skin, nice hair, good facial features, and a thin, fit body. Some of the major agencies have divisions that represent mature models.

Characters

Character models generally appear in print ads and television commercials. This type of model is one who can exhibit funny or bizarre characterizations. To get an idea as to the types used in this category, look through nonfashion magazines. You'll see gardeners, teachers, secretaries, corporate executives, waitresses, and doctors—all of whom have two things in common: They're "real-people" types," and they are models.

If you have a unique look or enjoy putting on various character faces, you might enjoy this type of work. It is a lot like acting without lines, so you need to be outgoing and feel very comfortable about yourself.

This market is also very trendy. In any given fashion season, major magazines might recruit the strangest-looking people they can find for fashion editorials or advertisements and will hire character models. So if your timing is right, who knows?

It can be difficult to earn a steady living as a character model, and for most, it turns out to be a fun, part-time job. There are a few models who earn a living in character print, but it is rare.

CHAPTER FOUR

Do You Have What It Takes?

"It's kind of fun to do the impossible. If you dream it, you can do it."
WALT DISNEY

*M*ost people don't look twice at models when they pass them on the street. For the most part, models are very tall, thin, and ordinary looking. They tend to wear trendy, casual clothes, little or no makeup, and usually their hair is pulled back. Photographers, makeup artists, and stylists blend their talents to create those amazing images that sell magazines and products.

You can have tremendous potential to model and not be able to launch a career. You could have all the physical requirements–perfect skin; well-defined features; long, thick hair; even test shots that prove tremendous photographic quality–and still not be able to make it. It takes a lot of courage to break into modeling, and although many people dream of such an opportunity, some lack the confidence to make the first step.

Some aspiring models do not have what it takes to turn that dream into reality. They are no different than those who dream of becoming actresses, musicians, or writers. Some turn thoughts into action; others do

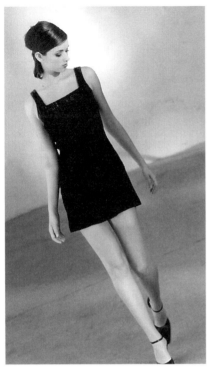

Kristina. Photo by Johnny Olsen. © 1999 Johnny Olsen Photography.

not. Whether it is low self-esteem or extreme shyness, most will stay in this dream mode as they go off and pursue some other means of earning a living. For whatever reason, they're never quite able to jump through the hoops, make the calls, and invest the time, energy, and resources to make their dreams come true.

A few are attracted to the modeling profession to obtain great photographs of themselves and capture their youth and beauty in print. Their main goal is to return home with a brag book to show friends, relatives, and future offspring how, once upon a time, they had entered the wonderful world of modeling. Without dedication and clearly defined goals, this type of individual will more than likely never ascend to a professional level.

Before setting off to pursue a modeling career, you should learn everything you can about what it is like to work as a model. You can get a step ahead of the game by reading this book, but you should also check out as many resources as possible and learn about the business before you make the decision to go for it. You should also be ready to make an honest personal assessment of your physical attributes, emotional stability, basic personality, and overall desire to succeed at a modeling career. Karl Rudisill, President and CEO of DICE, a digital composite company in New York, advises models to "Be honest with yourself. Be able to see yourself on the cover, or in the catalog—and if you can, then pursue your modeling career."

What Does It Take Physically?

I've already mentioned some of the attributes required to be a successful fashion model, and we are all exposed to pictures of perfect models on a daily basis. Most of the top agencies recruit models that fit specific physical requirements. The exceptions, of course, are those agencies that have divisions for other types, like plus–size models. Requirements can also vary in different geographic locations. In Miami, for instance, you could easily succeed if you are shorter than 5'8".

For the most part, models have similar characteristics and fit the standards issued by major agencies. But the fashion industry is notorious for quick changes and trends. It's common for a model to barely hold on for long periods of time, rarely getting bookings, and then all of the sudden (seemingly overnight) become extremely popular. One season you'll see magazines filled with blue–eyed blondes with perfect hair. The next year, quirky models with wild hair and less than perfect looks are in. It does no good to mention current trends, because by the time you read this, everything will have changed. In this business, timing is everything.

More than likely, you already have some idea of what type of modeling would currently suit you best. Now take a look at the requirements listed below, and think about where you might find a niche in the future.

New York Industry Standards

Since the heartbeat of the fashion industry is in New York City, clients in that market set most of the standards. New York is the place to make connections with top clients and get booked for prestigious magazine covers and editorials.

The industry standards regarding physical requirements are as follows:

- *Height:* As mentioned earlier, the ideal height is 5'9" and taller. According to Monique Pillard of Elite, "Being 5'9" is not as critical as it used to be–it has a lot more to do with personality." Although most models represented by top agencies are still 5'9" and up, Monique advises that a prospective model who is shorter will need to be very, very strong in other areas to be considered for representation. In general, advertising agents and photographers believe that long and lean is the most photogenic. Models also need to be the standard size, size 6 to 8, so that they can fit into a standard size of clothing. The preference is for the upper leg to be shorter than the

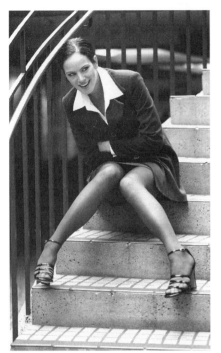

Photo by Chris Lawrence. © 1999 Chris Lawrence.

distance from the knee to the foot.

• *Body:* A long, lean, and toned body is essential. Most models end up shooting everything from lingerie to swimwear and usually show a lot of skin. Sometimes a girl who looks normal according to everyday standards is asked by an modeling agent to lose ten pounds before being considered for representation. To anyone else, the model may look perfectly fine and within the healthy weight standards for her height and frame, but in order to work as a model, she needs to be a standard size 6 to 8. It is rare for a straight-size fashion model to wear a size 10.

• *Posture:* A model should be able to walk, sit, stand, and move with confidence and grace.

• *Skin:* A model must have clear, beautiful skin free of blemishes, birthmarks, scars, or discolorations.

• *Teeth:* Straight, white teeth are essential.

• *Facial features:* Most models have distinct facial features with well-defined cheekbones; full, shapely lips; and widely spaced eyes.

• *Hair:* Shoulder-length hair is preferred, but all lengths of hair are acceptable. Hair should be healthy and natural looking.

• *Photogenic quality:* Most skills can be learned, but there's an undeniable, undefinable quality that successful models have. They don't freeze in front of the camera–they move with the mood and really come alive on film. Oddly enough, some extraordinarily attractive individuals do not photograph well.

• *Youth:* The preferred age to begin a modeling career is thirteen, with an upper range of twenty-two. Monique Pillard says, "There is no perfect age to start. We take models as young as thirteen to fourteen years old." Most agencies currently recruit very young models, and it is not unusual for a thirteen- or fourteen-year-old to have her modeling career in full swing. The majority express concern in taking models as young as Monique uses. Her reasoning is simple: "I personally don't like taking models that young, but in order to remain competitive, we do. If we don't take them at age thirteen, the agency down the street will."

These requirements are only a guideline. If you fit most or all of the above requirements and are photogenic, you are physically suited for modeling and could find success in this profession. But don't be discouraged if you don't measure up. There are still plenty of opportunities to be found in modeling if you have the desire to find out where you fit in. What are your best features? What market exists in your hometown? Are you willing to relocate?

Depending on your attributes and the level of passion you have to pursue this profession, some physical characteristics can be changed or improved. There are ways to improve your complexion or straighten your teeth. You can certainly lose excess weight, get in shape, improve your hair, or work on your poise. Although characteristics like height and bone structure can't be changed, things like skin discolorations or facial imperfections can be fixed by a good plastic surgeon. Before deciding what direction to take, make an honest assessment of your existing physical qualities. Next, make a list of things you believe you need to change in order to pursue a modeling career. Are you willing and able to do what it takes to make these physical changes?

Beyond Beauty

Beyond physical attributes, the important elements needed to be a successful model are things you can't see. In fact, most agency representatives look for attributes that are beyond physical beauty. An upbeat personality is one of the first things that catch their attention. Here are some other qualities that contribute to a successful modeling career:

Ambition

If you want a career in modeling, you should want it with such an intense burning desire that you are able to be rejected, criticized, and still believe in yourself, even through long periods without a booking. Your desire to succeed will be the fuel that provides you with the energy needed to keep moving forward. Maintaining that energy will help you remain optimistic in the face of rejection.

Attitude

A good attitude is imperative if you want a steady, successful career as a model. If you have negative thoughts about the professionals you work with, the designs you are wearing, your hair, makeup, or what you are asked to do, keep it to yourself (with due regard to personal safety, of course). If you strongly dislike the personalities of some of your coworkers, do not discuss it with others. Negative talk breeds more negative talk and brings everyone down. A positive person can bring everyone up, so if you are very upbeat, have a great sense of humor, and are ready and willing to work with all the professionals on the set, you'll develop a good reputation and be remembered. Photographer Pascal Preti advises models to "understand the fashion business and personalities in this business, be confident, and have a great attitude." Having a positive, cooperative, and professional attitude will get you booked again and again.

Communication

A professional model is one who can listen, understand directions, and provide the action required. D. Brian Nelson, a professional photographer based in southern California, advises models to "listen to what the photographer is saying and don't talk too much." He once worked with a model who kept interrupting his communication with her own suggestions and did not bother to fully listen to what he was trying to say. Like I said, he worked with this model *once*. You'll be asked to change your pose, move around, create a mood, and hold a position for a long time while literally hundreds of shots are taken. Photographers can become frustrated if a model can't follow directions or refuses to do so. Model Luria Petrucci advises, "The best models have the ability to understand what a photographer or art director wants. They reinvent themselves time and time again to produce outstanding results and great campaigns." So relax, listen carefully, focus on what you are doing, don't be afraid to try something new, and respond naturally.

Competition

If you look through magazine editorials, advertisements, or agency head books, you'll see hundreds of beautiful, perfect-looking models. Depending on the type of modeling you pursue, you'll also see these models at go-sees, castings, and at the agency. There will be models who are taller, younger, or more out-

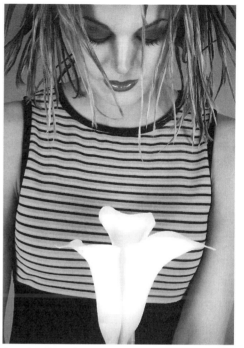

Photo © 1999 Andrei.

going than you are. Remember, you are unique, and your look will appeal to the right client for the right job. Competing for jobs is always going to be a part of what you do, so focus your attention on your own best attributes and abilities.

Confidence

At castings, you can find yourself in a room with fifty other models who are all after the same job. And this might be your tenth go-see in a week. You must be confident enough to not only handle rejection, but to also hold your head high and feel good about yourself. Kwok Kan Chan of Marilyn, Inc., told me that "confidence, energy, and personality" are the ingredients that catch his eye. Most agents look for these same traits. If you don't feel good about yourself, you're not going to be happy. And if you're not happy, the pursuit of a modeling career is not worth the trouble.

When you are starting out, as a model or in any other profession, it is normal to feel insecure. You are learning your craft and do not know what to expect, so sometimes you have to work a little harder at maintaining a high level of confidence.

Criticism

The modeling profession is notorious for being candid, brutally honest, and not always tactful. You might run into an agent who will tell you you'll never work as a model. Or, you could be hired to work on a shoot and have the photographer complain about the way you move. If you are able to listen, put your feelings aside, and give it all you've got, you'll get through the day a lot easier and might even learn something from the experience.

Often models in search of an agency will be told, bluntly, that they need to make a change. Maybe it's something easy to accomplish, like altering a hairstyle or losing ten pounds. As model Joanna Marie suggests, "You need to develop thick skin and realize that sometimes criticism is useful and delivered with the intention of helping you. Try not to take it personally. You must be a very strong person. Many people may turn you down for jobs or just be downright nasty, but as long as you have a good opinion of yourself, you'll be able to let it roll off your back and not take it to heart."

Listen to the advice professionals offer, evaluate their comments, and decide for yourself what you need to do (if anything) to make a change.

Determination

Do you usually get what you want once you set out to achieve a goal? Or do you think about it but easily become sidetracked or lose your motivation? In order to thrive as a model, determination is crucial. You must be able to go on castings when you're tired, fill your personal time with testings, and devote your energy to pursuing your career. Given the short life span of most models' careers, there's not a lot of room to slack off. Understand the downside and be willing to keep focused on where you want to be, not where you are now. The demands are great, and the modeling profession can be all consuming, but a successful career in modeling can be extremely rewarding.

Discipline

A model should be focused on her work and dedicated to her career. Day after day, you hit the pavement and sell yourself as a model. There's no room in this business for models who blow off appointments or stay out and party half the night away before a booking. Take care of yourself, treat your career like a business, and say no to tempting indulgences. Kwok Kan Chan of Marilyn, Inc., advises models to "Treat your modeling career like a business. Invest in yourself and your education–not just college programs, but try to take advantage of where this career can take you. You can travel the world. Try to see and enjoy some of the places you go when possible, and start developing your skill in investing your money."

Energy

To an outsider, it seems as if it would be so easy to stand in front of a camera or walk down a runway. The fact is, it can be exhausting. It takes a lot of energy to fill up a day going to go–sees, castings, testings, hair appointments, fittings, and actual bookings. Photo shoots can take a long time and are usually physically challenging as well. You don't just sit there and look pretty. It's more like stretch, hold the pose, stretch a little more, and hold that pose even though your back feels like it's breaking. The stress of performing on a runway, working in front of a camera, or interviewing for bookings can deplete energy. A busy modeling career is not for one who needs to indulge in a long, daily nap. Those who find success have plenty of energy to get them through.

Flexibility

A flexible, professional model is able to change directions halfway through a shoot. This model will always give 100 percent and has a reputation for being both cooperative and professional. Modeling can be grueling work, not at all glamorous, and sometimes not even fun. You might feel completely stupid in the outfit you are wearing. You might feel crazy in the way you are directed to move in front of the camera. Learn to set your personal feelings aside and do everything you can to work within your environment. If you are wearing something you wouldn't be caught dead in on the street, wear it, work with it, and make it feel and look like it's the most sensational garment you've ever seen.

Independence

Most beginning models who are sent to Europe have never previously been far from home, much less out of the country. Suddenly, they find themselves in a foreign land with neither friends nor family nearby. Home-sickness is difficult enough to deal with, on top of finding your way around and living amongst people who speak with heavy accents, if they speak English at all.

The modeling life can be lonely. You will make new friends, but once you start becoming successful you'll find that you have a minimum amount of social time to devote to cultivating relationships. You might have a social engagement planned and find that you have an early-morning booking the next day.

Even if you don't end up going out of the United States, moving to a major city can be almost as difficult an adjustment. Think about the following questions and answer them honestly:

- Are you independent enough to handle being on your own?
- Are you willing to find solutions to problems on your own?
- Does the thought of traveling and being around people you don't know for months at a time make you nervous or excited?
- How dependent are you on your friends and family?
- Do you place a great deal of importance on what others think of you?
- Do you feel good enough about yourself to not let it bother you if your friends or associates find fault with you?

On a positive note, the independent lifestyle gained through modeling can be very rewarding. For example, take Stephanie Averill, who has been modeling for a number of years and never has a break in her schedule unless she decides to "book out." Stephanie has always used her time wisely—on and off the set—to read, learn, and continue to cultivate her personal interests and education. "Models need more balance in other areas of their lives," she explained, "because there's so much time spent on having to look at yourself, one can start to get too critical."

Jealousy

Sometimes a young model finds herself far removed from the environment in which she grew up, and her new lifestyle is often envied by friends and family members. Often it is hard for friends to understand or relate to one who travels to exotic places, appears in national print, and earns a great deal of money. Especially if said friends are still at home, flipping burgers at the local fast-food restaurant. As model Leslie Adair explains, "No one who 'knew you when' can understand this life. You really can't expect them to. They don't understand why you just can't do the things you used to do. Friendships are built on commonalities, and when that changes, the friendships change." Jealousy can creep into relationships, and suddenly you find that those whom you thought were your friends are not. Are you emotionally ready to take this type of rejection?

Money Management

Can you manage your money? If you have just earned $1,200 for a booking but don't have anything else lined up for the month, would you (a) take some time off, (b) buy some clothes and makeup, or (c) put the money toward your expenses and save what you can for leaner times? If you are starting out, you'd better think of the leaner times, because when you're new, bookings don't happen every day.

If you've been working for six months and find that you are earning several thousand per week, would you (a) get out of the model's apartment and find a place of your own, (b) hit your favorite designer boutiques, or (c) spend moderately and save your money? There's no right or wrong answer here, but as you might guess, the wisest thing to do is to start saving. This will help you get through the leaner times and serve as an investment in your future. You might not be modeling five years from now, and if you've saved or invested part of your earnings, you could take time off to complete your education or start your own business.

Your ability to save and plan ahead might enable you to pursue dreams beyond modeling.

Patience

For most models, success does not happen overnight. You have to be willing to work hard and be patient. Karl Rudisill of DICE recommends, "Don't give up too soon." Karl, who modeled for Ford before becoming a photographer, was about to "cash it in" when, all of a sudden, his career took off. He shared another story with me about a male model he knew in Europe who was struggling. The model was below the standard height, so Karl recommended that he go to Japan. His career took off instantly—he found enormous success in the Asian market.

From the moment you sign with an agency, you'll be testing, waiting for your prints, putting together your composite, and lining up at go-sees. Even when you begin to work, you'll often have to wait for everything to come together on a shoot. Sometimes technical things go wrong and it takes more time than planned. You have to develop a great attitude and learn to be very patient and flexible.

You should also be prepared for the inevitable downtime you'll experience. It can be a little unsettling not to know when you'll work again, particularly in the beginning. If you are the type of individual who needs the security of a steady paycheck, this may not be a good profession for you. Be patient, have some means of financial support other than modeling (at least at first), and maintain a high level of self-confidence.

Organization

Since a model's life is in a perpetual state of movement, she must be prepared for everything from packing the right items needed for a shoot to planning her day so that she can feasibly get from place to place without being late. This requires an individual who is willing and able to organize and plan ahead.

Details are crucial: what's needed on a shoot, clear directions to where a casting call is located, and what you need to bring along to the job. You won't have a successful go-see if you forget to keep enough composites in your book—the last thing you want is to not be able to leave a card at an appointment. If you forget to write down an important casting call, you've missed an opportunity. If you've booked too many calls and there's no possible way to get from one to the next on time, you're blowing your credibility by not showing up or arriving too late. You might need an extra pair of stockings on a shoot, or a different pair of shoes. In modeling, your calendar is your lifeline, and it must be maintained accurately. If you're not that organized now, ask yourself if you're willing to make organization and attention to detail a part of your everyday life.

Other Interests

The perception in the modeling business is that most models, even those who have become successful, are not happy. Those models who do appear to be happy have one thing in common: They maintain their own interests outside of the modeling business. For example, Christy Turlington pursued her college education and, in 1999, earned a degree in liberal arts from Boston University. Several well-known models have written books. Padma Lakshmi, an internationally known print and runway model, wrote *Easy Exotic: A Model's Low-Fat Recipes from Around the World*. Maintaining other interests–other than fashion–seems to be a key trait in those who have enjoyed long, satisfying careers.

Perseverance

As long as modeling is something you believe you can do, you need to be determined not to give up. Will you stick to it, weather the storms of rejection, and refuse to throw in the towel? It's common for models to finally find success just when they are about to go back home. All of a sudden, the heavens part, and they start to get work. Model Danielle Peterson recommends, "Never give up. 'No' comes a lot more often than 'yes' does."

Personality

Put yourself in the place of the casting agent. Image you've narrowed your search down to two models. Based on the two composites you've seen, they are both equally suitable for the booking. You bring in the first model. She looks around the room, barely makes eye contact with you, and hands you her portfolio. She seems confident and very proud of her look but just sits quietly as you examine her book. She sits very straight, on the edge of the chair, and seems very polished. You've barely seen her smile, and what few questions you've asked are met with very brief "yes" or "no" answers. Sure, she's gorgeous and looks great in print, but you get the feeling she's not someone with whom you'd want to go have a cup of coffee.

Now you're ready to see the second model. She walks in with confidence and smiles warmly as she enters the room. She extends her hand and makes eye contact. She is polite, warm, and friendly. She is proud to show you her book and answers your questions with enthusiasm, giving you details. There's a sparkle in her eyes, and you get the feeling this model would be a gem to work with–easy to direct and flexible enough to create the images your client needs. Which model would you hire? Which model would you be at the casting?

Professionalism

In any profession, reputation is important. There are many models competing for the same job, and professionalism is one area than helps set them apart. If a client has to choose between a model who is known to throw tantrums and is notoriously late and a model who is always on time, cooperative, and pleasant to work with, it's not hard to figure out which one gets the job. Be honest, develop a good business sense, and always conduct yourself in a professional manner.

Your professionalism may sometimes be challenged by the personalities you encounter. Sometimes things go wrong on the set. There's a lot of money on the line, as well as the reputations of the professionals you work with, and tempers can flair. Patience runs out. Fuses blow. A true professional remains calm and does not let the temperament of others throw her off balance.

Rejection

You might think you are the next Cindy Crawford until you walk into a waiting room at a go–see and find that it's filled with thirty other models who look just as good as you do. If you don't find ways to deal with rejection, modeling can be a miserable career. It is a known fact that you are not going to be right for every job that you seek. You have to be able to handle continuous rejection and not let it destroy your enthusiasm or self-esteem. Accept this fact before you begin a modeling career and prepare yourself by knowing that rejection is a big part of the business.

Modeling, at times, can be a brutally honest business. In other words, you might go out on a go-see and have a client make an opinionated evaluation about your looks. For instance, "Your lips are too big." A model has to be able to shrug off negative information. At the next go-see you might hear, "Your lips are perfect!" Remember, it's all relative.

Resources

It takes time for most models to start earning a living in this profession. The overnight sensation is very rare, so you need resources to fall back on. How much do you have in savings? Do your parents support you financially? Are they willing to continue supporting you while you try to get your modeling career off the ground? If not, do you have skills to work part-time, if need be?

Strength

Are you strong enough to say "no" to drugs, drinking, or staying out partying all night? If you want to succeed as a model and have a long, healthy career, learn to resist temptation. There's no room in this business for dark circles under the eyes, low energy, or altered moods. Drugs, alcohol, and sleep deprivation affect looks and personality—and looks and personality are what you're selling.

Vision

Look ahead and think about your life beyond modeling. Kwok of Marilyn, Inc., advises models to "Use this opportunity to observe what everyone else is doing. You might want to consider photography, or other professions, when finished with modeling." If you are still in school, can you balance this career with the demands of continuing your education? There are ways to work as a model without sacrificing your degree. If you start to work on a steady basis, ask your agent about professional study programs. There are also unconventional ways to get an education, including online degree programs where you can complete your course work via the Internet. If you travel with a laptop computer, you can pursue your education on your own time. Although you might be busy with travel, castings, appointments, etc., you'll find plenty of downtime on the set or on an airplane to study. Don't lose sight of things you want to do after your modeling career is over.

A novice model needs to learn how to change the way she views herself. Her looks, attitude, and the way she presents herself are her commodity. When you sit down to review your test shots, you should be able to look at them objectively. Some models fall in love with their work, but others want to pick themselves apart. When you review your work, don't be overly critical. Learn to view your photographs objectively, as a product.

Weight

How sensitive are you about your weight? If an agent told you that you need to lose ten pounds, would you be willing to lose weight in order to model? Frequently, models are turned away by agents who ask them to take off a few pounds and then come back. Many don't come back. Models have to learn to eat a balanced diet to maintain energy and health without putting on excess weight.

All the inner qualities described in this chapter are important if you want to pursue a modeling life. Still, models complain about constantly being judged by their looks. It isn't easy to be physically evaluated every day without much consideration for who you are inside, but it's certainly a part of being a competitive model. Once you get tear sheets in your portfolio and start to work more steadily, the game will change, and you'll find that you're judged more by the work you've produced than by your looks. An upbeat, organized approach will definitely help you get the work and build that portfolio.

CHAPTER FIVE

Creating Your Image

"Beauty is in the eye of the beholder."
MARGARET WOLFE HUNGERFORD, IRISH WRITER

*I*f you haven't been one to study fashion, keep up with trends, designers, photographers, top models, magazines, and all that pertains to the world of fashion, now is the time to start. Since it can be expensive to go out and buy an armful of fashion magazines, you can easily get what you need by investigating other resources. Your local library has a wealth of information. Invest a few hours and browse through magazines. Pay attention to what type of models are being used, how they look in print, and what expressions or emotions they portray. Be aware of the names of photographers, makeup artists, designers, and other professionals represented.

Another great resource is the Internet. You can browse through an endless number of Web sites that contain the latest fashions, trends, designers, models, agencies, etc. If you don't have access to the Internet, go to your local library. Some colleges also have computer labs or other resources that provide Internet access. If you are not familiar with comput-

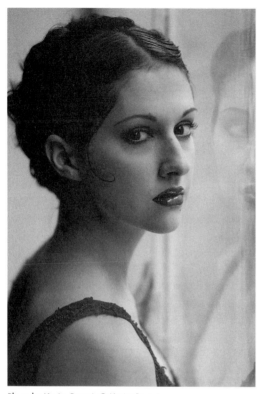

Photo by Karim Ramzi. © Karim Ramzi.

ers, see if you can find a basic computer course offered through a community college. Usually, these classes are very affordable, and you'll walk away with the ability to research anything you want.

Study fashion trends, know what designers are popular, and gain a sense of what types of clothing they create. Soon you'll start to develop your own style as a result of doing your homework.

In fact, one of the greatest benefits of modeling experience is a better self-image. A model must continuously work on creating and presenting a strong image. Some models who have been at it for a while claim this is one of the things they dislike most about the profession–having to constantly look their best without allowing as much as a nick in their nail polish. The residence where I lived in New York was filled with models and actresses who were trying to get their careers off the ground. In fact, we'd often get together to network and share stories of our various successes and failures. One particular model was given the nickname "Prissy," but she was actually one of the few who enjoyed regular bookings. However, she always complained the loudest about having to maintain her beauty routine. "It's not that I want to let myself go," she'd say, "but occasionally it would be nice to not have to constantly worry about such superficial stuff–like hair, makeup, and wardrobe." Of course, I don't think any of us ever saw Prissy having a bad hair day.

The fact is, the competition is so fierce, you must continuously work on your image if you want to succeed. Think of your modeling career as a business and your image and personality as your greatest assets. Whether it's finding the perfect hairstyle, learning how to apply makeup like a professional, or keeping a fit and toned body, the model's image must be strong to compete. That doesn't mean you have to get rid of everything commonly considered to be a flaw. Remember, some imperfections can be very distinctive, like Cindy Crawford's mole.

It is your job as a model to learn everything you can about taking care of yourself from top to bottom. A wealth of information is

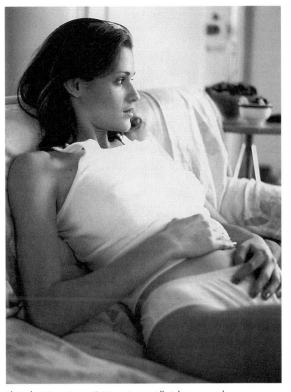

available on the Internet, and you can't pick up a woman's magazine without seeing articles on beauty, fashion, and physical and mental fitness. (Books are a great resource, too, and you'll find several recommended in chapter 20.)

If you sign a contract with an agency, you should receive some instruction on basic grooming. You'll also learn a lot from the makeup artists and hair stylists you will work with on testings and bookings. Your sense of fashion and the development of your own style will begin to evolve when you start to work as a model.

The ideas presented in this chapter are basic. I strongly recommend you read some of the books on skin care and makeup (listed in chapter 20). If possible, invest in professional makeup lessons, manicures, and pedicures. As long as you continue to model, you will need to explore beauty basics, self-care, and the elements that help create your image.

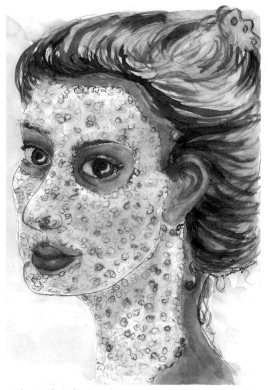

Art by Nicole Nolasco.

Basic Skin Care

A model's skin will go through a lot on a typical work day (for example, heavy makeup, exposure to weather during photo shoots, working under hot lights, and so on). Most makeup and skin–care professionals recommend that you use good, natural–based products. The basics are: cleanser, toner, moisturizer, and an exfoliating or a deep–cleaning mask.

Always start with a clean face before applying makeup, and develop a skin–care regimen to be performed before going to bed each night. Don't neglect your neck. When you're young, it's easy to overlook your neck, but unfortunately, it's one of the first places that begins to show age.

Invest in a good makeup–removal cream. Select a cream that can also be used to remove eye makeup and mascara. Gently apply the cream to your face and eyelashes and remove it with a warm washcloth.

Exfoliation is a very important part of your skin–care regimen. On a regular basis, you need to rid yourself of dead skin cells, which will help promote new cell growth and give you a healthy glow. If your skin tends to be dry and flaky, it could simply be because of a buildup of dead cells. Sometimes makeup remover does not deep–clean your face and remove these, which causes your skin to look flaky.

There are plenty of exfoliating products on the market, or you can experiment with natural, homemade products. One I have tried is an oatmeal and yogurt facial–scrub mix. If your skin is dry, try this one: In a small bowl, combine one tablespoon of olive oil with two tablespoons of oatmeal and two tablespoons of plain yogurt. Mix the ingredients well, then massage into your face and neck. After a few minutes, rinse off with warm water, followed by cold water. If you do not have dry skin, you might want to try the mixture without the oil.

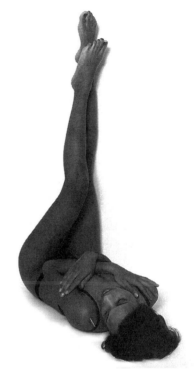

After exfoliation, you should use a toner to remove excess oil from your skin. Toner is very refreshing and leaves your face feeling cool and clean. In hot weather, try storing your toner in the refrigerator.

Moisturizer is an important part of your skin-care regimen. Find a moisturizer that will work with your skin type and not leave your skin feeling oily. Avoid moisturizers or any products that contain alcohol. Those products tend to dry out your skin. Massage the moisturizer into

Photo by Chris Lawrence. © 1999 Chris Lawrence.

the face and neck area. If your skin is very oily, you might not need to use a moisturizer every day.

Avoid foods and situations that cause breakouts, if you are prone to this type of skin problem. If you break out easily, you might also want to try using a nonalkaline or medicated soap.

Body Care

There are great bath products on the market, from wonderful bath oils to exfoliating scrub creams. Make sure you use products that do not dry out your skin. Your moisturizing lotion is very important. Apply it generously after your shower or bath.

Massage is great for increasing circulation, working the soreness out of muscles, improving your skin tone, and relieving stress. If you ever

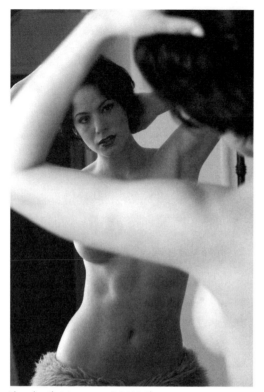

Photo by Chris Lawrence. © 1999 Chris Lawrence.

really want to treat yourself, try an hour with a masseuse. Swedish massage is a deep, relaxing massage that eases muscle tension. Shiatsu is a Japanese massage technique that uses finger pressure in order to release energy flow.

Always wear sunblock on your face and body. You should repeat the application every few hours if you are in the sun all day. Don't forget to apply sunblock during the winter or on overcast days—you can suffer from sunburn on cloudy days, too.

Self-tanning products have come a long way. I remember using them as a majorette in high school. The cream had a distinct odor, and if you weren't careful, you'd end up with orange streaks. You still have to be careful and apply the product evenly so that it will not streak your skin, but fortunately, the results are a lot more natural looking (and smell better, too).

Posture

Often, tall girls have to learn the art of good posture. When teens grow taller than their peers, they often slump their shoulders. It's as if they try to slink down to an average size so that they won't feel like giraffes. By learning to sit up straight, you'll look more confident and be more noticeable.

To make sure your shoulders are in the right position, put your hands on your shoulders and roll your arms back. That's where your shoulders should remain. After you roll your shoulders back, put your arms to your side. Bend your elbows, then place a broomstick straight across the small of your back, holding the broomstick in the crooks of your elbows. I know this sounds odd. You'll probably feel like a Barbie doll at first—but once you relax and the position becomes natural, your body will look elegant as you walk down the runway. Don't be surprised if these exercises feel strange—people slump most of the time and feel odd when they hold their bodies in the proper position.

Nail Care

To learn how to take care of your nails, have a manicure and pay attention to what the professional does. To do your own manicure, you will need:

- Base coat
- Cotton balls
- Cuticle remover
- Cuticle trimmer
- Emery board
- Hand cream
- Nail buffer
- Nail polish
- Nail polish remover (acetone-free)
- Nail strengthener
- Orange stick
- Q-tips
- Small bowl of warm, soapy water
- Top coat
- Towel

Remove all of your nail polish. Use a Q-tip to get into the corners if you have difficulty removing your polish. File your nails using an emery board. Soak your hands in warm water with a mild soap or oil (you can use a bath oil) for a couple of minutes. If your skin is sensitive to nail-care products, soaking your hands for up to five minutes could help

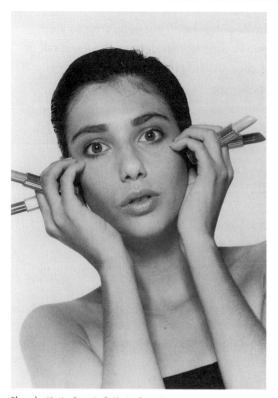

Photo by Karim Ramzi. © Karim Ramzi.

counteract the effects of the chemicals in the polish remover. Massage hand cream into your hands and remove the excess lotion from your nails. Push back your cuticles with an orange stick and apply cuticle remover, if necessary. Trim the cuticles and buff your nails. Apply a nail strengthener, especially if your nails are prone to splitting or breaking. Apply a base coat, allowing each coat to thoroughly dry. Apply your shade of nail polish. Do not use more than two coats of polish. Make sure each coat completely dries between applications. Apply a top coat. It is very important to do your manicure when you have plenty of time and are not rushed in any way. You should always choose neutral and natural-looking colors that will work with anything you model.

While there are many methods and products available to fix a broken nail, you might want to try the "tea bag" method. It's quick, easy, and usually long lasting. Remove all nail polish and clean and buff your nails (even the broken nail). Cut a small piece of material off a tea bag (enough to cover the nail tear) and set it aside. Using your emery board, lightly stroke the broken or torn nail area to roughen up the surface. Carefully apply a tiny drop of Super glue on the broken nail and place the tea bag snippet over the area. Allow this to dry, then cut away the excess mesh. Take the emery board and lightly file down the tea bag portion, blending it with your nail. Buff the nail and apply a good base coat, then continue your polish regimen. One word of caution: Be extremely careful using this type of glue. It dries fast and can literally glue your skin together. Also, avoid the cuticle area to cut down on the risk of a nail infection. This method works best when used on a nail that is slightly torn on the side, but is not totally severed.

Feet

Models are on their feet for long periods of time, running from go-sees to bookings or working in heels on the runway for hours. Protect your feet by wearing comfortable shoes while going from appointment to appointment.

Treat yourself to a pedicure and pay attention to everything the professional does to your feet. This is how you should be taking care of them on a regular basis.

Soak your feet in warm water mixed with your favorite oil or bath product. Use a pumice stone to smooth out or remove dry skin. After cutting your nails, smooth them out with an emery board. With a Q-tip, push back the cuticle and continue to massage the oil into your feet.

Dental Care

Naturally, you should keep up with regular dental appointments to maintain healthy teeth. But as a model, your smile needs to be particularly bright. There are many products on the market for teeth whitening, and the cost of professional bleaching is fairly reasonable and can be done in approximately two to three weeks. The laser whitening method can yield results in one appointment, but if your funds are limited, you might want to try an over-the-counter teeth-whitening product. Rapid White Tooth Whitening System is a product that is endorsed by model Kim Alexis. The kit comes with a conditioning prewhitening toothpaste, the whitening gel (which is placed in a plastic mouthpiece), and a finishing rinse. The taste is slightly unpleasant after you remove the mouthpiece, but it's a small price to pay if you get results.

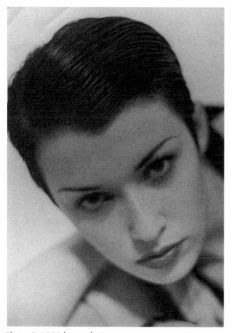

Photo © 1999 by Andrei.

Makeup

One of the best investments a model can make is professional makeup lessons. In one lesson, you can learn all about the art of contouring, what your best colors are, and some tips for photographic makeup. A great place to go in New York is Makeup For Ever Professional, a SoHo boutique located at 409 West Broadway; (212) 941–9337. If you don't have access to a professional makeup artist, there are several books on the art of applying makeup. (See chapter 20 for more information.)

A Model's Makeup Kit

A model must always have on hand the products and tools needed to apply professional makeup. A makeup kit should contain:

- Blush powder or cream, various shades
- Contour powder
- Cosmetic sponges
- Cotton balls
- Eye shadows in a variety of matte shades
- Eyebrow brush
- Eye drops
- Eyelash curler
- Eyeliner pencil
- Eyeliner powder
- Foundation

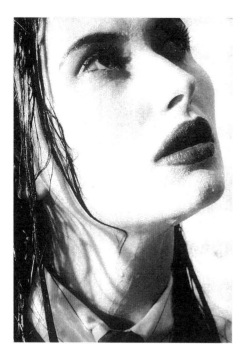

Photo © 1999 by Andrei.

- Lip gloss
- Lip liner pencil, various shades
- Lipstick, various shades
- Makeup remover
- Makeup brushes for application of translucent powder, blush, eyeliner, contouring powders, lip color, and eye shadows
- Makeup mirror
- Mascara
- Moisturizer
- Q-tips
- Tissues
- Translucent powder
- Tweezers

Basic Makeup Skills

Most models wear little, if any, makeup. But even if you don't wear much makeup, you need to know how to apply it like a professional. (Makeup application for photography is a little different than everyday makeup; that technique is covered in chapter 8.)

Invest in a good, natural–looking foundation. The purpose of using foundation is to even out your skin tone. Your foundation should blend with your skin tone and match perfectly. Blend foundation to your jaw line. Do not apply foundation to your neck.

If you have dark circles under your eyes, or any skin discolorations, a concealer might be necessary and should be applied before using foundation. Translucent powder is used to set your makeup and should be used after your highlighter, blush, and eye shadow. Apply powder with a powder brush, shaking off excess powder before application.

When applying makeup, use downward strokes across your nose, cheeks, and chin area and upward strokes around your eyes. Apply foundation to the entire face, even the eyelids. If you want a lighter, sheer look for daytime, apply your makeup by using a cosmetic sponge. In the summer, if your foundation is water–based, you can use a small amount of cold water on the sponge to achieve an extremely sheer, natural look.

Purchase a good, full brush to apply powder blusher. Apply directly

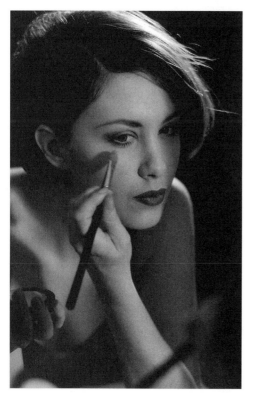

Photo by Karim Ramzi. © Karim Ramzi.

on the cheekbone area (the apple of the cheek) using an upward motion. Blend blush by using a cosmetic sponge or tissue by softly rubbing the edges of where you've applied the blush. The intention is not to have a hard line, but to have the color blend into the face.

In the daytime, you will probably not need to use eye shadow. But for special occasions or at night, you can have fun with the application of more color. Apply a light, neutral shade to the entire eye area from the brow to the lid. Use a darker shade to contour the crease of the eye. Basic matte earth-tone colors are best. To apply eyeliner, experiment with an eye pencil as well as powder liners applied with a special eyeliner brush.

Use a Q-tip or cosmetic sponge to blend eyeliner. If a product causes a reaction, such as a sty on your eyelid or itchiness around your lashes, throw away your mascara and eyeliner and purchase new products. Eye makeup can become contaminated, and you don't want to continue to infect your eyes.

Curl lashes with an eyelash curler. Be sure to keep your lash curler clean; if too much mascara residue builds up on it, the lashes could stick to the curler. Apply mascara to lower lashes, then upper lashes. For day-time use, you will probably only need one coat of mascara. For evening wear, apply two to three coats of mascara, allowing each coat to dry between applications.

Professional artists spend a lot of time, often up to thirty minutes, just blending eye makeup, cheek contour powder, and blush. So take your time, experiment, and learn what looks best on you.

With a large sable brush, apply loose translucent powder over the entire face, including your eyes. Be sure to shake off excess powder before applying. Too much powder on the face gives the appearance of wearing too much makeup and can emphasize small lines and wrinkles.

Keep your lips moisturized, and line them with a lip pencil or lip brush. Apply lip color, then blot with a tissue. If you are wearing a light shade of lipstick or a gloss, you will not need to line your lips.

Hair Care

A model's hair generally takes a beating. When your hair is curled with hot rollers, teased, sprayed, and pulled up and torn down to create a look—on a daily basis—your hair will need extra attention. Conditioning with an intensive treatment at least once a week can help keep hair in good condition. Nutrients such as vitamin E and cod liver oil can also help keep hair healthy.

When it comes to deciding how long or short your hair should be, take a look at the models you admire in magazines and catalogs. Often an agency will advise you on what to do to update your look, but you should always use your own judgment as well. You might want to consider a longer hairstyle because of versatility. It can be put up in a French twist, braided, curled, or worn straight. No matter what type of hairstyle you end up with, experiment with different ways to style it. In some fashion shoots, you need to be able to change hairstyles just like you change outfits.

If you want long hair, you might consider hair extensions. Great Lengths is a hair–bonding system that fuses real human hair to a client's existing hair. Extensions can be natural looking, easy to manage, and a great way to instantly get a head of long, thick hair.

Models are notorious for coloring their hair. There are many products on the market that are economical and easy to use. If you are experimenting with a new color, try a colored mousse that can be washed out, or a temporary color. If you are using a permanent hair color, be sure to do a strand test and follow the directions carefully.

If you have access to a computer, you might want to take a look at a

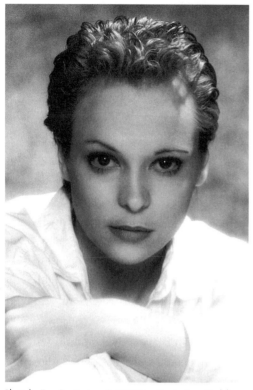

Photo by Tom Farrington. © 1999 Tom Farrington. Model: Danielle Peterson.

program called Cosmopolitan Virtual Makeover. By scanning in a photograph of yourself, or having your film processed onto a disk or CD–ROM, you can choose from hundreds of hairstyles and makeup options on your computer. This software program is available in most computer stores and is a great way to preview new looks without suffering from a bad haircut or color choice.

Overall Health

In order to keep up with the fast–paced life of a model, you need to maintain good health. Your health is a reflection of general well–being. Diet and consumption are important, but other factors such as sleep, stress level, and physical fitness also are important factors.

Sleep

Getting enough sleep is critical for maintaining healthy skin. During sleep, your body rids itself of toxins. Premature aging and dark circles under your eyes are the results of sleep deprivation. Most people need at least eight hours of sleep in order to maintain health and well–being.

Combating Stress

A model's life is filled with factors that can cause a great deal of stress. Life can quickly become unbalanced when the demands seem greater than your ability to keep up with them. Another stress–creating factor is change. The modeling industry itself is in a state of continuous change, and when a model starts out, her whole life changes. It is not the changes themselves that cause the problems; it is the way the model reacts to them.

What physically happens when you are on stress overload? Adrenaline is released into the bloodstream, preparing an individual for "fight or flight." This natural mechanism helps us cope with dangerous situations or shock. When stress is prolonged, though, it can cause various health problems, like frequent headaches, muscle tension, or exhaustion.

The biggest reason to combat stress is the toll it can take on your appearance, which happens to be your most important asset. You can probably determine what generally creates stress, but it's important to recognize and write down exactly what fuels your own personal stress. Next, think about how you react to those things you've listed. Is there a way to turn your negative reactions into positive ones? How many things on the list do you actually have control over? Learn to accept things you cannot control, and appreciate the learning experience you gain from them. Then put things into perspective and ask yourself this question: In the grand scheme of things, how important are these things, anyway? What's the worst thing that can happen? Usually, it isn't as bad as you've built it up to be. Here are a few more ideas to help you combat stress:

- Get organized so you won't spend your time searching for things.
- Exercise.
- Laugh out loud.
- Vent your feelings when you need to.
- Try yoga or meditation.
- Try an Epsom salt bath, which has the benefit of drawing toxins from your body and easing muscle tension.
- Do something nice for someone else. (This one is my favorite–it really works!)

Exercise

Models are known for their beautiful bodies, and they do everything from rigorous fitness routines to yoga to keep in shape. Most of them are involved in several physical activities that help them maintain their per-

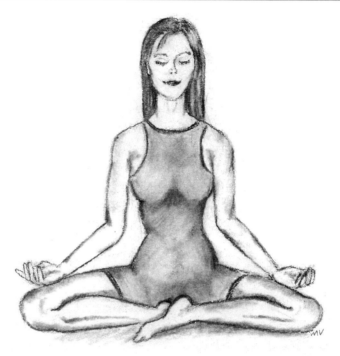

Sketch by Maria Vasseur.

fect bodies, like running, swimming, walking, kickboxing, and dancing. At one time or another, most models have worked with a personal trainer. Since models maintain tight schedules and travel extensively, it's good to establish a fitness routine that can be maintained while on the road. Most models interviewed for this book highly recommend yoga as a great way to stay fit. Model Leslie Adair agrees: "Yoga keeps your body toned, limber, and helps with jet lag and mental focus."

Nutrition

One of the best things you can do for yourself as a model (and as a person!) is learn as much as you can about nutrition. Since modeling is a profession that centers around thinness, there is a tendency to skip meals and crash diet. This type of behavior can wreck your health over a period of time. One of the most noticeable things it can do is slow down your metabolism and reduce your energy level. Models need plenty of energy, and your diet should provide all the nutrients your body needs to sustain good health. Your daily food consumption should include protein, carbohydrates, fats, and fiber.

If you don't get enough B vitamins, you can become depressed, nervous, or cranky. Iron deficiencies can cause forgetfulness. Thiamin can help you feel calmer and rest better, and B–12 gives you energy.

Carbohydrates have a tendency to calm you down and provide energy. Sugar and caffeine can make you feel jumpy and stressed.

Drink six to eight glasses of water a day. Water is vital for keeping your skin healthy by flushing toxins and waste through your body. Carry around a water bottle with you at all times and make drinking water a part of your everyday life. Soon, you might find that you prefer water over other beverages.

Don't smoke. If you do smoke, try to quit. Not only does smoking age your skin prematurely, it robs your body of vitamins B and C. Cigarette smoke carries toxins in the bloodstream and restricts blood flow to the skin, which causes aging and diminishes the skin's natural healthy glow. Cigarette smoke also lingers on your skin, breath, and clothing, which can be a turn–off.

Weight Loss

Although you might walk into an agency fitting into a size 8, you could still be required to lose a few pounds. The request to lose weight is very typical for models trying to get established with an agency, so don't be shocked if it happens to you. If you've never had to deal with losing weight before, the best and most sound advice is to follow a healthy eating program and exercise. Far too often, models resort to the latest fad diet, fasting, or other unhealthy approaches to losing weight, and most who do will eventually gain those pounds back or struggle to maintain the weight loss they've suffered to achieve.

A healthy approach to weight loss is to eat vegetables, fruits, whole grains, low–fat or nonfat dairy products, and lean meats such as chicken or fish. Don't skip meals; it can lead to overeating and slow down your metabolism.

In order to lose weight, you should engage in at least thirty minutes of activity for three to five days per week. Combine aerobics, walking, dancing, kickboxing, or whatever activity you enjoy most, but make sure you choose something that will accelerate your heart rate for the duration of the activity.

Developing Your Own Style

Most models dress casually for go–sees and castings. You should be comfortable, but wear clothing that emphasizes your figure. Short skirts are fine, or tight leggings. Styles will continuously change, so keep up with the trends and select things that make you feel comfortable and confident.

Whatever you do, don't get overly serious about any of this. A great attitude can compensate for many, many physical shortcomings.

CHAPTER SIX

Finding the Right Agency

*"I know the price of success: dedication, hard work, and an
unremitting devotion to things you want to see happen."*

FRANK LLOYD WRIGHT

*I*f you live near one of the major mod-
eling markets, there are specific guidelines that will help you find representation. The smaller markets are more flexible and varied in the way
they do business. However, before you start seeking an agency to represent you, do your homework. Make sure you have read chapter 10, Avoiding the Dark Side of the Business, before you choose an agency. It could
save you a lot of heartache, headache, and money.

Small-Town Realities

Can you get started in modeling if you (a) live where there are no major
agencies and (b) you're not quite ready to move to a major metropolitan
area? Yes is the correct answer to both questions, but you'll have to do a
lot of self-promotion, and you must be extremely proactive. If you live in
a small town, there are two different ways to launch a modeling career

without relocating to a major market: local modeling and registering with a model management company.

Local Modeling

Some small towns with no modeling agencies nevertheless have plenty of department stores, boutiques, and newspapers with local advertisements. You can go to your local department stores or dress shops and ask if they participate in fashion shows or local advertising. Let them know you are interested in modeling. If you have put together a portfolio (see chapter 8), go further: Tell them you're a model. You can also check with charity organizations to see if they sponsor events or fashion shows that utilize models. If you have access to a well-known, reputable photographer, get in touch with him and ask if he uses models and if he will consider you. Make a list of contacts that might utilize you as a model. Does the local women's club conduct fashion shows? If not, you might suggest one as a fundraiser. Finally, check with your local newspaper. Often, local papers do fashion editorials–things like bridal, back-to-school, or seasonal layouts. If you want to model on a local level and there's no agency to represent you, this is the easiest way to get started.

While pursuing modeling on a local level may be fun and adventurous, it is highly unlikely you'll be able to earn a living at it. Think of the experience as a test run, which will help you determine whether you want to pursue modeling as a career.

Model Management Companies

Another way to model without moving to a major market is to register with a model management company that represents models from diverse geographical areas. A great agency on the West Coast that represents models in the international market is Model Management International. This management company is very reputable and has a very professional, high-quality listing of models. Check them out at *www.modelmgmt.com*.

Go International is another example. This agency is located in Columbus, Ohio, and has a solid presence on the Internet (*http://go-international.com*). Mona Overton and Kathy Robertson have recruited models from all over the country, booked them for jobs in the international marketplace, and helped them land contracts with modeling agencies. Go International Model Management, Inc., is located at 2151 East Dublin-Granville Road, Suite #216, Columbus, OH 43229; (614) 882-9010. You can also contact them through their Web page or mail a snapshot to them–no matter where you live.

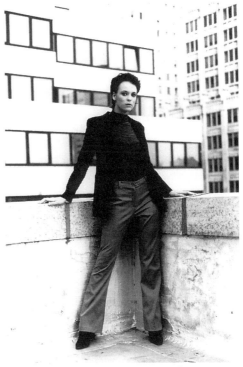

Photo by Stephen Clark. New York City Rooftop. © 1999 Stephen Clark. Model: Danielle Peterson. Makeup: PBSC Inhouse.

Average-Size Cities Outside the Major Markets

If you live in an average-size town but are still outside of the major markets, you'll probably find a few agencies or even modeling schools. Follow the same guidelines in investigating these businesses as you would any other. Additionally, you will want to find out what type of fees the agent charges for placing you, how much work is available, and what you might expect to earn. Smaller markets are typically great for getting a start and finding out a little more about the industry, but in order to turn modeling into a career, you need to focus on the larger markets. There are extensive lists of agencies located in most cities across the United States, which are easily obtained from a variety of sources (see chapter 20 for more information.)

Major Markets

If you live near a major city, like New York, Miami, Chicago, or Los Angeles, approach a top, well-known agency first. The feedback you receive will be valuable. I met with David Vando of Models Mart in New York briefly; he advises models to be patient and adds, "Conventions are one way to see agents in or near their own town, but yes . . . they can do the same thing in New York on their own. Another possibility is to go to other markets in cities like Chicago, Miami, or Los Angeles."

You can learn whether you have what it takes to model for a major agency. Top agents might point you toward a smaller agency. If they don't express immediate interest in you, ask them what you need to change in order to attract their attention. (A list of agencies located in the major metropolitan areas is listed in chapter 19.)

Tips for Finding an Agency

Find out what agencies are located in your hometown or in a nearby city. Make a list of the agencies you want to consider, with their telephone numbers, addresses, and any information readily available. Be prepared to call them to confirm the information or to fill in gaps in information you need. You need to find out:

- Are they accepting new models?
- What are their requirements (type, size, height)?
- Do they have an open call?
- If so, on what days and at what time?
- If not, what is their process? (Send in photos by mail?)
- What is the address? (Be sure to confirm the address if you plan to visit.)

Don't be timid about calling agencies. They get calls from many hopeful models who, like yourself, seek information. Obtain as much information as possible about the agents before you meet with them. Keep track of who you have seen. If you plan to visit several agencies, it will probably be helpful to write down your impressions and the agency's feedback as soon as you leave the appointment. Go have a soda or cup of coffee and write down your ideas while they're fresh in your mind. This is particularly valuable if you are seeing several agencies in one day. It will help you keep your perspective, remember your options, and narrow down your search.

Most agencies have a certain overall "look," and it would be to your benefit to find out what your potential agency's look is all about. If the agency has a Web site, take a look at the models it represents and see how you'd fit in. Try to be objective, and don't be intimidated.

Most agencies offer an "open call," which is a set period of time when new models are interviewed. You don't need an appointment to interview during an open call, but you should find out what the agency's requirements are. In other words, if you are a full-figure model, make sure the agency has a full-figure division.

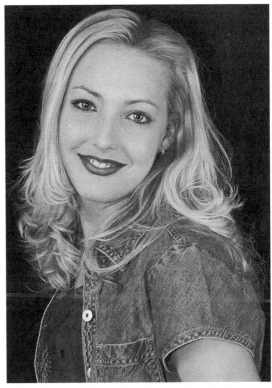

Shonna. Photography by Bradley Charles Herlein. © 1998 MODEL-LIGHT.com.

If you are 5'5" and the height requirement is 5'9", don't waste your own or the agent's time. Find an agency that represents your type, and make sure you meet its requirements before you show up for an interview.

Not all agencies offer open calls. Most agencies (even if they have open calls) prefer to receive photographs of a model through the mail. They're not looking for glamour shots or pictures that resemble a shot from *Vogue*–they want very basic photographs: one of your face, or a headshot, and one full-body shot. Have a friend or parent shoot a few rolls of film and select a couple of the photos to send to the agent. Keep it simple; no overdone makeup, fancy hairdos, prom-queen photos, etc. Just a clean, simple, natural-looking representation of what you look like is all that's needed.

Make sure your photographs have labels on the back with your name, address, and telephone number. You should include a basic letter expressing your interest in the agency, indicating that you are available to meet with agents at their convenience. Be sure to thank the agency for its consideration—good etiquette can mean a lot. Include your statistics (i.e., height, size, eye color, hair color, age) in the letter, along with your return address and current telephone number.

If you want your photographs back, send a self-addressed, stamped envelope for the agency's convenience. If you are sending photographs to several agencies, you might want to select your two best photographs and have copies made. Reprints are relatively inexpensive and, in most places, can be obtained in a few days or even overnight.

Please do research on any agency that is not familiar to you. Oja Fin, from The Model's Guild, suggests, "Don't be afraid to follow your true instincts . . . if something doesn't seem right, leave."

Pay attention to agents' feedback. If they say that you're not tall enough, you can ask them if there is any category in which you could work, perhaps with another agency. Or ask them if they can recommend another agency for which you might be more suitable. If you've seen several agencies and they all say the same thing, you should consult as many people as possible for opinions on how you can find your own niche in modeling.

After your first interview, an agency may not give you a firm commitment. The agent might ask to see you again. This doesn't necessarily mean that the company is not interested, but for various reasons, it might not presently be able to sign you. The agency could have too many of your "type" under contract or might want to see you after you've had a haircut and lost ten pounds.

When I set out to pursue modeling, I took one week off and went to New York to visit agencies. I didn't have any appointments lined up, but I had my heart set on visiting Ford. On my first day in the city, I called Ford to find out if they had an open call or if I could get an appointment to see an agent. I was told no, that I had to submit a snapshot first, and then Ford would get back to me. I dropped off an envelope the next day; it contained a couple of pictures and a note with my physical statistics. I left the envelope with the receptionist at the Ford office and hoped I'd get a call at my hotel during the week. I didn't get the call, but a few weeks later, at home, I received a handwritten letter that said, "Thank you for your interest in Ford. While we can make no commitments at this time, we will be happy to set up an appointment to see you in January. Please call us once you have moved here."

I was thrilled to find that the Ford agency wanted me to come back. That was all the encouragement I needed to make my move to New York City. But even after I had moved to New York, it still took several months before Ford could see me. The letter indicated they would be ready to see me in January, but it was months after I had moved before I could get in to see them. I didn't know it at the time, but one of the major plus–size agencies was closing, and Ford was about to take on a lot of its models. Finding an agency is often a very frustrating process–especially when you can't wait to get started.

Learn to use your judgment when it comes to feedback from agencies. The agency's advice might not be right for you. You have to trust your instinct. Take a look at the role models: Lauren Hutton was told to get her teeth fixed; she chose not to and became a tremendous success. Cindy Crawford followed the same path with her famous trademark mole. Some–times, not looking completely perfect makes you stand out from the masses.

A prime example of differences in what an agency expects when con–sidering a new model is the issue of a portfolio. Depending on where you live, an agency might expect to see a portfolio when you meet with them for the first time. If you're in New York and meeting with top agencies, they will probably not even look at your book. Instead, they'll want to see your fresh face without much makeup and will look at a snapshot or take a Polaroid. They want to look at you as an artist would look at a blank canvas in order to visualize what they might be able to create.

If you have a set appointment with an agency, be on time! Just like interviewing for a job, being late leaves a bad first impression.

Sometimes a model will start out at a smaller (also known as a "bou–tique") agency to get her foot in the door. Then, once the model starts working and gaining recognition, one of the big agencies will more than likely start knocking on her door to steal her away. This is not unique to modeling–it happens frequently in many areas of the entertainment business. Although it is naturally preferable to stay with your agents if they're working hard for you and getting you bookings, sometimes the grass looks greener in the bigger meadow, and successful models make a switch, thinking the larger agency can serve them better. Oftentimes, the competing agency will try to negotiate a lower commission, which could make the offer seem even more appealing. This may be tempting, but keep in mind that a good, strong relationship with an agent who is booking plenty of work with top clients may be better than signing with a larger agency. You might remember that old Southern maxim: "If it ain't broke, don't fix it!"

Interview Questions

Before you start meeting with prospective agencies, outline what you want to find out and prepare a list of questions to ask. Don't be shy or embarrassed to query the agent representative. Some new models feel they don't know enough about this business to ask questions, yet there are things they really need to know. Here some suggested questions with which to start:

- Do you expect all models to sign a contract? If so, what are the terms? How long of a commitment do you require? Do you ever represent models without a contract?
- What is the agency's commission rate and how is it paid? Is it the standard 20 percent? Is it deducted from the model's pay?
- For what expenses is the model responsible?
- Does the agency use headshots or publish an agency book? If the latter, how often? At what time of the year? What is the cost?
- What is the agency's payment policy? Do clients have to pay the agency before the model gets paid? (Models who work with reputable agencies receive payment on a regular basis, even if the client has not paid the agency for the model's services.)

Unknown Agencies

New agencies crop up all the time. Sometimes a fading agency will assume another name in an attempt to create a new image or will be bought out by another agency. If the agency in question is not familiar to you, investigate it thoroughly. Once you have read chapter 10, you will have a good idea of the potential pitfalls and scams that exist, but here are a few tips for checking out an unknown agency:

- Take a friend with you, preferably one who does not want to model and who really does not have the right look to model. See what the agents tell your friend. If they seem interested in her and tell her the same thing they told you, then you'd better watch out, particularly if they ask for money.
- If you are asked to purchase a portfolio with the agency's photographer(s), be wary.
- Don't feel pressured into signing a contract. If they are interested in you today, they will probably be interested tomorrow. Ask to take a copy of the contract home to review. This is a very reasonable and intelligent request.
- Don't buy into an agency that wants to charge you money for classes or training. The exception is a modeling school that also serves as an agency. Even then, the cost of training should be minimal.
- Remember, one big warning sign is when an agency tells you that you'll get a lot of work or make a lot of money. Although reputable agencies know the types of models they can market, there's no guarantee that you will get work. You will be competing with a lot of very beautiful, talented models. The only thing you have as a guarantee (other than physical attractiveness) is your confidence in yourself and a burning desire to make it happen.
- Last but not least, go with your gut instinct and don't ignore the warning signs.

It is doubtful that you'll be perfect for every agency you visit. If an agent tells you your look is not right, don't give up. There have been plenty of models who were turned down by one or more agencies who went on to find one that would work for them. Learn to take rejection in stride and move on.

CHAPTER SEVEN

All About Agencies

"Follow your bliss. Find where it is and don't be afraid to follow it."
JOSEPH CAMPBELL

For some models, signing a contract with one of the large, well-known agencies is a one-way ticket to success. Most people have heard of the agencies Elite, Ford, and Wilhelmina, which have signed several top celebrity models. In response to the recent trend of actresses gracing the covers of popular magazines, some of these agencies now represent famous film stars for print work.

There are hundreds of modeling agencies across the United States, with the majority found in major cities such as New York, Miami, Chicago, Dallas, and Los Angeles. There are also agencies in San Francisco, Boston, Seattle, and Washington, D.C., and if you care to investigate further, you'll discover that many small towns across the country have agencies. The question is, do they have a lot of work for models?

Although there are no set rules or regulations for agencies, you'll find that most of them operate in a similar manner. There may, however, be some differences in how an agency in Iowa operates versus one in New

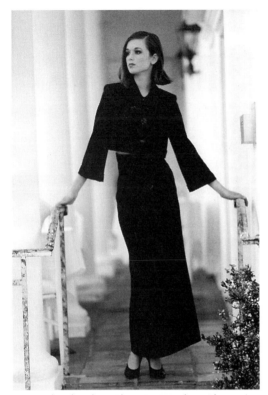

Kristina. Photo by Johnny Olsen. © 1999 Johnny Olsen Photography.

York. This chapter focuses on the operations of larger agencies in major markets, so keep that in mind if you compare this to what is available in your hometown.

What Does a Modeling Agency Do?

It is rare for a model to work on a freelance basis; successful career models work through agencies. An agency functions like an employment agency, obtaining work for models by providing models for clients. The agency charges a fee for its services, both to the model and the client. The industry standard is 20 percent from the model and 20 percent from the client, although occasionally other terms are agreed upon. Reputable agencies do not charge a model a fee to join the agency or to get started. The 20 percent commission is taken out of the model's pay after she earns money from a modeling assignment. When a model agrees to be represented by an agency, she typically signs a contract and agrees to obtain modeling assignments through the agency. That agreement does not include agencies she will work with outside the city or country; the agency will coordinate those arrangements and work out the terms.

Model Management Companies

To gain access to professional agencies all over the world, get representation through a major agency (like Elite), or directly book international assignments, a management company may be a good first option. Because of the international contacts some management companies have, models can receive extended assignments, sometimes for several months, in countries like Japan, Taiwan, or Korea. Since some of these firms serve international clients, their requirements can vary and be a little less strict than a high-fashion agency in one of the major U.S. markets. For example, a 5'7" model could work very well in the Asian market.

As mentioned previously, management companies often help models link up with major agencies. When the management company places a model with a modeling agency, the management company will continue to claim a percentage of the model's fees for a designated period of time. These details are ironed out between the management company and the model's new agency.

The management company operates as a "mother agency" for the model and can help the model narrow down her search for an agency in a major market as well as prepare the model for agency representation. (For more information regarding model management companies, see chapter 20.)

Agency Professionals

President/Director

The agency's president or director is responsible for the type of models the agency represents (high fashion, commercial, full figure, teens, children, men). The president builds relationships with clients and the media and serves as the primary spokesperson for the agency as well as oversees the hiring of staff and all other interworkings of the agency. If the agency is large and represents different types of models, there will be a director for each division.

Agent/Booker

A model agent is commonly referred to as a *booker*. Your booker/agent will become one of the most important people in your career. If you sign with an established, reputable agency, the agents will take you under their wing, groom you, and promote you in the areas in which they think you are most marketable. They will be the liaison between you and your clients–you are not responsible for contacting clients for work.

Your agent will help set you up with photographers for testings. The beginning model may work with several testing photographers before she has enough prints suitable for a portfolio and composite card. The agent will then work with the model to review the photographs and select the strongest shots for the composite card and portfolio. After the portfolio is put together, the agent will use the composites to promote the model, sending cards out to prospective clients. The model will also be sent out on go–sees, which are appointments established for the model to "go see" clients.

Your agent will schedule or book modeling jobs, negotiate fees, and work out all the specific details. Once you start working, she will keep track of prints from magazines and catalogs that you have appeared in (tear sheets) and help reorganize your portfolio.

If a model is sent outside the United States, the agent serves as the liaison between agents that represent the model in cities in foreign countries. While such international relationships are usually worked out over years and foreign agents can be trusted, if questions or problems arise while you are working outside the United States, you can always contact your home–based or "mother" agent for advice and direction.

~

Your Relationship with Your Agent

Since your agent is the most important person in your career, build a strong, solid foundation from the beginning. It is crucial to develop a sound relationship with your agent based on mutual trust and understanding. Talk over anything you are not certain about. Don't be timid about asking questions or letting your agent know when something is wrong. When you are starting out in any profession, there is much to learn— modeling is no different. Your agent is the primary source for information.

Your agent should always be available to help solve problems that occur on bookings. That doesn't mean that every time you break a nail, you call your agent. Be respectful and cognizant of your agent's time and don't waste it for anything that isn't truly important. Keep an open line of communication with your agent and be patient and understanding when you're not first on his list. Agents have other models to work with as well, and they juggle a lot of things at once. The inner workings of a busy agency are intense and highly stressful, so always be patient, professional, and respectful of your agent's time.

Depending on the agency, you might have one agent that you work with, or several. In smaller, boutique-type agencies, since agents represent fewer models than the larger, well-known agencies, the model will establish working relationships with all the agents, and each one will know everything needed to promote the individual model. Some models report more individual attention in a smaller agency as opposed to "getting lost" in a larger agency. It totally depends on the model, what her needs are, and how comfortable she is with the agency. That's why it is important to meet with several agencies before you decide which one best suits your needs. I enjoyed meeting with various agents in New York and was amazed at how different each and every one was, from the different personalities of the agents themselves to the general atmosphere at the agency. Kwok Kan Chan of Marilyn, Inc., advised that a model should "feel comfortable about the environment of the agency and feel a connection with the agents." It makes perfect sense, too; after you've seen a few agencies and can witness firsthand just how different they can be, you'll instantly know which agencies feel like home.

You will be expected to call your agent on a daily basis (usually at the end of the day) to find out if you have go-sees, get details on bookings, and get general feedback from your appointments or actual jobs. Your agent will let you know when you should call, and you should never neglect to do so.

You should have complete confidence in your agent's ability to manage your career, trust in your agent's knowledge of the market, and listen to her suggestions and advice. If your relationship with your agent is not on this level, then you need to consider whether you need to find a new agent.

~

Accounting Personnel

Most agencies employ an individual (or several individuals, depending on the size of the agency) to handle accounting matters. This includes the expenses incurred by the agency, the billing of clients, payroll, keeping up with the models' ledgers, and complying with contract details and bonus payments from clients.

Public Relations

If the agency is large and well known, a public-relations professional is typically hired to maintain its image and reputation. This function is particularly important to models when magazines, newspapers, and television programs what to know more about them.

Support Staff

Like most businesses, agencies hire secretaries to assist the director(s), prepare or write communication, organize materials and contact information, answer telephone calls, and generally help with the overall operation of the business. A large agency will employ a receptionist, who provides the primary contact with models, photographers, clients, editors, media professionals, and the general public. At a large agency, the flow of telephone calls is enormous, and the receptionist is simultaneously responsible for meeting and greeting important clients, new models, and other professionals visiting the agency. Needless to say, the receptionist plays a vital role in maintaining a smooth-running agency; the visitor's first impression of the agency often comes from the receptionist.

Because of the large volume of photographs, composites, and portfolios that need to be instantly transported across town to clients, magazine editors, or photographers, most large agencies hire messengers. Messengers are responsible for getting a model's portfolio from client to photographer and back to the agency quickly and efficiently.

All of the professionals who work within an agency are generally very hard working and dedicated. It takes a very energetic, bright individual to keep up with this fast-paced business, and each professional is an integral cog in the wheel that makes the agency machine run smoothly. If you recognize how important these individuals are and always treat them with the utmost respect, they will continue to go that extra mile for you.

The Test Board

If you join a larger agency, you will probably start out in an agency's "new faces" division or "test board." This is where the new model focuses on testing with photographers, building a portfolio and composite, and gaining responses from clients. This gives the agency the opportunity to see how to best market the model, and it gives the model a sample of the business, so she can determine whether she wants to continue to pursue modeling as a career. Sometimes a prospective model is put on the test board before the agency formally agrees to represent her, reserving the right to see how the model moves and looks in print before making a commitment.

Agencies and Housing

Most reputable agencies help new models find housing by setting them up in models' apartments. These apartments are leased by the agencies, which rent the rooms to models on a weekly basis. Models' apartments vary from brownstones to doorman buildings. These accommodations are similar to a college dormitory setting in that a model will share a room with other models. Karen Lee, who chaperones Elite's apartments, says the apartments are clean, safe places for models to stay. "There are rules in the apartments, such as no boys, no drugs, and no alcohol," Karen indicated, "but staying in the apartment will give new models the opportunity to meet other models."

Travel and Relocation

Occasionally, an agency will pay for airfare for a prospective model to relocate, and even for a parent to accompany her if she has tremendous potential. Again, it depends on the model, her economic situation, and the agency's belief in her marketability. If the model decides to sign a contract with the agency, she is often put up in a models' apartment, and the rent is also advanced until she starts to get bookings and earn money. The same advancement of travel and living expenses is applicable when an agent sends a new model to Europe. This is, again, deducted from the model's earnings. It is not something that is to be expected, however. Whether an agency advances money for you to relocate, or even for travel to meet them, depends on many factors, so don't be disappointed if you are not offered such an arrangement. It could merely be an issue of timing. While you may have been signed if you were already relocated, the agency might not want to risk investing money up front when it already has several models of your type.

If you are sent to Europe, you will more than likely work with several agencies during your stay. You will have duplicate portfolios at those agencies, and they will be responsible for sending you out on go–sees, testings, and bookings. Your "mother" agency, or the agency who sent you, will remain your main point of contact.

A model can work for several agencies in various cities and countries around the world, but only one main agency in the city where she begins her career. In other words, if a model signs a contract with Elite New York, she might have ten other agencies she works with in Paris, Milan, Germany, and Switzerland. Elite New York will still remain her "mother" agency. If a model is brought in by a smaller agency–in Kansas, perhaps– and ends up signing a contract with Elite New York, Elite becomes her "managing mother agency" to agents in foreign markets. The agencies involved work out commission agreements with one another. It is not the responsibility or concern of the model to be involved in this negotia- tion process.

The Contract

Most contracts vary in length of time commitment from one year to sev- eral years. An agency can sign one model for a single year and then sign the next model for three years. Even within an agency, there are no set rules. (More information regarding contracts is provided in chapter 14.)

Promotion

An agent frequently interviews new photographers who are interested in testing models. After testing, the agent will select photographs from the test session that can be used in the model's portfolio. After a model appears in print (catalog or magazine), the agent will obtain copies of the magazine and gather the tear sheets for the model's portfolio. Most agents know precisely what images to use in putting together the model's portfolio and composite card. They know the market and what their clients want to see and can select the proper images from the model's photographs and tear sheets.

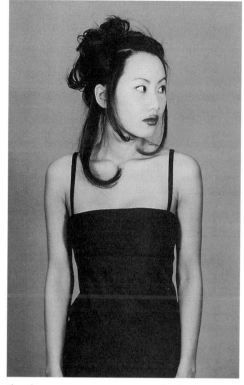

Large agencies usually produce a promotional book on an annual basis, and some agencies produce a poster or head sheet. A promotional book contains photographs of all models the agency represents. Often, two to three body shots and a head sheet are included for each model, along with her name and statistics. A "head sheet" is just as it sounds—a sheet that contains a headshot of each model. These promotional materials are sent out to clients, editors, designers, and photographers—the industry professionals who hire models.

Finding New Models

Agencies recruit new models in numerous ways. In addition to the open calls and photo submissions discussed in the previous chapter, most agencies "scout" for models, and some employ professional scouts. Scouts often use simple, straightforward methods to find new talent, and some have even been known to walk the streets with a Polaroid camera ready to recruit models. For example, Charles Short, from Aline Souliers Management, prefers to scout from the street. "I like to find models who are not desperately seeking this profession–those who hadn't really considered it, yet have the potential." Charles looks for those who have the standard model traits, but beyond beauty, those who exhibit a good attitude and have personality. Scouts approach individuals whom they feel might have model potential at the supermarket, at the airport, or in a restaurant. They give the prospective model the agency's credentials and leave it up to them to follow up.

Some models are found through model management companies or conventions. There are a few reputable conventions that travel across the United States, giving prospective models a chance to learn more about the business and meet industry professionals. A modeling scout for an agency or agent will attend conventions in hopes of finding a new face, but, according to most agents, it is rare to find a model with potential at a convention. (For more information about conventions, see chapter 18.)

Contests are another way agencies find models. These competitions are advertised in magazines, and information about them is also available on the Internet. Some agencies, like Elite and Wilhelmina, host annual events. ModelNews.com hosts a "Model of the Month" contest where the winner goes to Los Angeles, California, all expenses paid, to meet with some of the biggest West Coast agencies. Finalists in other competitions are typically flown to New York, all expenses paid, to compete for contracts and prizes. Most contests will guarantee modeling contracts, along with very attractive prizes, to the lucky winners. For example, Wilhelmina's event for February 2000 offered a Wilhelmina modeling contract valued at $50,000 as First Grand Prize along with an editorial spread in *Essence* magazine. Recently, *Mode* magazine and Wilhelmina teamed up to sponsor a modeling contest for their full-figure division. Keep your eyes open for contests–it never hurts to submit an entry. Usually the prizes are terrific, and the opportunity to land a contract is certainly worthwhile.

Money Matters

There are no set standards in the modeling industry regarding what expenses models are expected to pay up front. Most agencies advance costs to models for travel and relocation, testing, and various other expenses. It all depends on the agency and its belief in the model's potential.

Before you meet with agencies, you should know how finances are handled and what the typical costs are in the business. New York is the main market in fashion, so the following information is specifically geared to this market. You will find, however, that the standards set in New York are also standard in cities like Miami, Chicago, Dallas, and Los Angeles.

If you decide to sign a contract with an agency, you need to have a complete understanding of the types of expenses you will be expected to reimburse. Be very clear about these details before you enter into any agreement so there will be no surprises.

Depending on a model's economic situation, expenses are often paid for or advanced when an agency is very interested in representing the model. If expenses are advanced, they are expected to be reimbursed after the model starts earning money. Standard expenses incurred by a model that will be paid up front or later deducted from her earnings are:

- Testings with photographers, which can cost anywhere from $25 (cost of film/printing) to $300.
- Portfolio books. Two to three books are often kept at the agency, and duplicate books are sent to other agencies with which you work.
- Composite card printing.
- Copies of prints or tear sheets for all portfolio books.
- Cost of copies of magazines that contain tear sheets.
- Model's bag (see chapter 9, "Things You Will Need").
- Makeup.
- Messenger costs, for when your book is sent to clients, photographers, etc.
- Fax costs, when information or prints are sent via fax.
- Replacement of composites and portfolio. (Usually, your card/book will be replaced every three to six months.)

- Modeling-agency book, headsheet, or poster.
- Travel expenses. Most of the time the client pays for airfare, but not always. This could be a potential cost to the model.
- Passport.

The agency maintains a ledger for each model, which reflects the monthly expenses incurred. Expenses, along with the 20 percent that goes to the agency, are deducted from her earnings. Since a model is considered to be an independent contractor, taxes and insurance are not deducted from her earnings—she is responsible for maintaining her business records and paying taxes.

If a new model decides she does not want to pursue this career and wants out of her contract, she could be liable for outstanding expenses. Any new model should have a complete understanding with the agency about expenses and termination arrangements before signing a contract.

Most agencies do not charge the model for:

- Registration fee or any type of "get-started" fee
- Expensive portfolio work with a designated photographer ($1,000 and up)
- Classes or training

Some schools serve as agencies in smaller markets, and you might find that classes or training fees are a part of what they charge. It is understandable that a lot of models want to get started in or near their hometown, so don't be put off by a local company's way of doing things. Just make sure you do your homework, investigate the agency's reputation, and find out if models actually get work after completing the recommended courses before you agree to the terms.

CHAPTER EIGHT

Building Your Portfolio

*"The people who get on in this world are the people who get up
and look for the circumstances they want and, if they can't find
them, make them."*

GEORGE BERNARD SHAW

$\mathcal{M}$ost new models get a little nervous
the first time they get in front of a camera. It seems like it would be easy
enough to pose, but modeling requires a lot more than just sitting or
standing there while the photographer snaps your picture. You have to
learn to relax, move with confidence, and be natural in front of a camera,
which usually takes practice to master. A model must be able to work
with the photographer, understand and conceptualize what is wanted,
and help create that mood. As editorial photographer Pascal Preti of 212
Artist Representatives, Inc. puts it, "Models must be flexible and able to
work with the photographer and crew to produce the shots they need. If
a model has a bad attitude, it makes the photographer's job more difficult,
and he will not want to work with her again."

Working in front of the camera requires the model to communicate
directly with the photographer through the camera lens, bringing creativity and spontaneity to the session. This is a fine art. As photographer

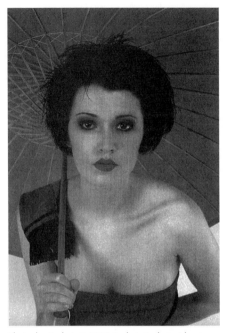

Karim Ramzi explains, "Each photographer has a different style, and no one can know how his creative process works and how he expresses his artistic abilities. The model should listen and follow his direction." The photographer gives the model an idea as to what type of images are wanted. Once the model starts to move, the session takes on a life of its own. The photographer begins to pull strong images from the model, inspiring the direction of the shoot. The photographer's enthusiasm energizes the model, the model's enthusiasm inspires the photographer, and the creative process moves to a whole new level. This communication between the model and photographer can be like a well-orchestrated dance, with both forces coming together to create outstanding images.

Photos by Andrei. © 1999 Andrei. Andrei wishes to dedicate these images to the loving memory of Brook Johnson, talented makeup artist and dear friend.

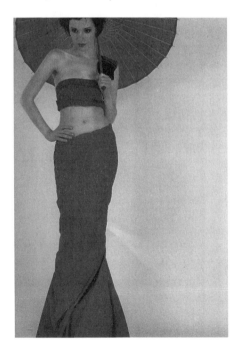

~

A Practical Miracle

A wonderful example of this creative process and the need for a model to be flexible and in total communication with the photographer is the fashion shoot that took place to capture the image below.

Johnny Olsen, a fashion photographer based out of Los Angeles, shot this image using natural

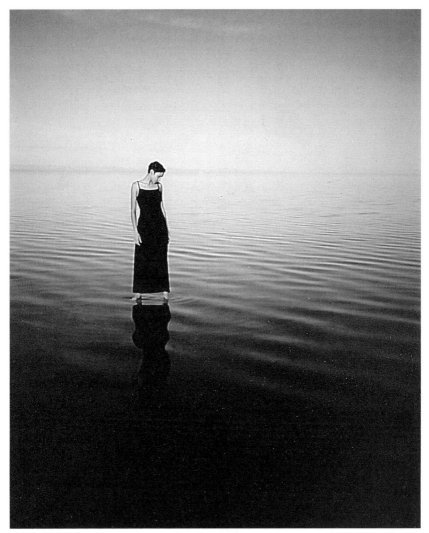

Photo by Johnny Olsen. © 1999 Johnny Olsen Photography.

light in the Sultan Seas. Although the setting looks soothing and exotic, the land was filled with dead fish bones, which carried an unbelievable stench. Johnny used several crates to build a stand beneath the water so that the model could pose on top, creating the illusion of walking on water. The model was placed on top of the crates, where she stood for several hours. She never complained as she worked with Johnny—and the results, this magnificent photograph, are clear. Oddly enough, while this entire shoot

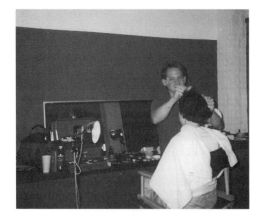

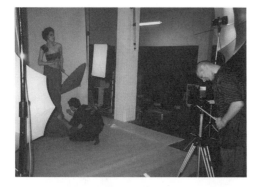

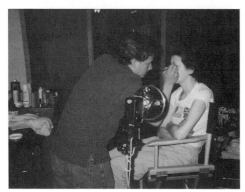

All photos, this and facing page by Andrei. © 1999 Andrei.

was taking place, the crew's vehicle was stuck in the sand—but this professional team decided to do what they came there to do—capture this image, which was inspired by the photographer. "I don't try to fix the results," Johnny adds, "I can go with a vision, and it's great when it just happens—the chemistry on the set and this synergistic effect."

Posing

So where do you start when you've never worked in front of a camera? Look at what others have done and at the composites of professional models. You will find plenty of agencies on the Internet, with more being added every day, that post composites and sometimes portfolios of models. Look at the Web sites of top agencies and see what types of shots really catch your attention.

You can also get a wealth of ideas from looking through magazines. Start your own tear sheet collection of ideas that you might want to try. You should look through every fashion magazine you can get your hands on. What types of mod-

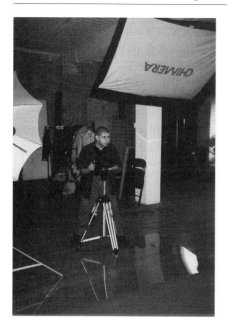
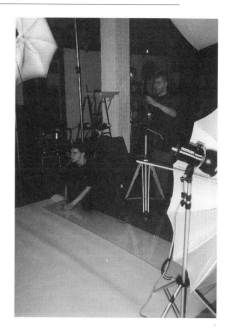

els are used? What do the models look like? What types of editorials catch your attention? How about advertisements? Take a look at the models' hair and makeup. Pay attention to who shot the ad or editorial. It's time to start becoming familiar with the artists who produce work. Who knows? You might be working with them sooner than you think.

Create a file folder and fill it with print work you admire, poses that catch your attention, and styles you can envision yourself wearing. When you're ready to do a practice shoot in front of your mirror, grab your file for ideas. Don't feel silly or vain standing in front of your mirror trying to replicate the poses you've pulled from other models. "Always avoid fake poses," advises photographer Karim Ramzi. "Be natural . . . do not put your hands inside your hair or twist your body thinking you will look sexy doing so . . . I would never use a model that would not be herself." Think of it as an actor rehearsing lines for a play. Examine your face and see what angles are most flattering. Practice different expressions or emotions. The more you practice, the more comfortable you'll feel when you do your first shoot. This exercise will give you an idea as to what looks best on you and will help you get used to moving and posing in front of a camera.

When a model is new, nervous, and unsure of how to move, the ten-

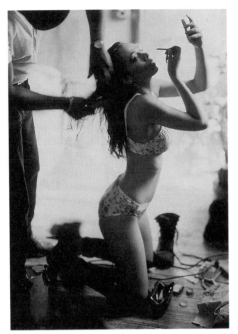

Photo by dr. wood. © 1999 dr. wood.

dency is to move too quickly. When you are just starting out, one of the most important things to remember about posing is to move in slow motion. The photographer might ask you to turn to the right, and if you move too fast, he could miss the best angles. In any given shoot, no matter what you are wearing, you can try different moods. Don't be shy about being sexy, happy, sad, angry, or shy during your tests. The photographer will be able to explore a variety of shots when you are willing to try different things, and there's a better chance you'll both hit upon something that works.

After the film from your testing session has been developed, the photographer will supply you with contact sheets, which contain all the shots from the roll of film, usually on an 8" × 10" sheet. You should invest in a loupe, which is a magnifying device used to view the small prints on the contact sheet. You should also invest in a grease pencil, available in most art-supply stores. You can use this writing instrument to draw or mark directly on the contact sheet, and you can remove the markings if you need to make changes in your selection.

One of the benefits of examining your contact sheets after a testing is to learn what worked well in the shoot and what failed. As you continue to test, you will become more comfortable and should soon be able to see improvement in your sessions.

Makeup for the Camera

Another element to preparing for a photo shoot is practicing makeup application. Applying makeup for print work is a little different than applying everyday makeup. Particularly when you start out, you should try to invest in having your hair and makeup professionally done. Ask your agency, other models, or the photographer you plan to work with for suggestions on hair and makeup professionals.

Some professional makeup artists offer personal consultations, or a one-on-one opportunity to learn how to apply your makeup professionally. This is well worth the investment, as most models need to know how to apply their own makeup with skill. If you do not have access to a professional, there are several books on the market that would be well worth the investment (see chapter 20).

A model must invest in a good makeup product line that is suitable for photography. Powder blush and eye-shadow products should be matte. Makeup products that shimmer and shine might be in style for street wear, but not for photo makeup. The photographer's lights will pick up those sparkles, and the effects are undesirable. You will also need several professional makeup brushes. Sable brushes are the most durable and practical for a model's use. It is worth the extra investment to have brushes that will last a long time and not shed. The basic makeup tools you will need are:

- Extra-large brush for powder
- Large brush for blush
- Several small eye-shadow brushes
- Eyeliner brush
- Lipliner brush
- Eyelash curler
- Eyebrow brush

If you do not have access to a good, professional product line, investigate Makeup For Ever's products (see chapter 20).

If you are responsible for your own makeup on a shoot, start with a totally clean, fresh face. Remove all makeup, including mascara, and apply a light moisturizer.

~

Advice from a Makeup Pro

Makeup artist Carole Weamer of Los Angeles offers the following advice:

- Be on time.
- Be rested.
- Always remove your makeup before going to bed.
- Get regular facials, manicures, and pedicures as well as professional eyebrow grooming and conditioning treatments for your hair.
- Don't be a diva.
- Be comfortable with yourself, move naturally, and enjoy your work.
- Wear sunscreen.
- If you have a product that you can't live without, bring it. It's OK to ask a makeup artist to use your own moisturizer, foundation, mascara, etc.
- You are the model. You don't have to like the clothes or the makeup, the client does. Wear the look gracefully. Complaining about the look will not get you hired again.
- Come to a photo shoot with clean skin.
- Don't have tan lines.
- Pay attention to fashion and makeup trends.
- Always use moisturizer, even if you have oily skin.
- Keep your makeup brushes clean; the colors will go on better.
- Don't use a powder puff for a long period of time; bacteria will settle into it, even if you wash it. They are inexpensive enough, so use one a week (the big peach ones).
- When you can, pay a professional makeup artist to do your makeup. It makes a *huge* difference.

~

Depending on your skin type, you may need concealer to even your skin tone, cover dark circles under your eyes, or hide imperfections. Use a sponge or your finger to apply the concealer to the dark areas of your face, then blend. One of the most important aspects of achieving photo–quality makeup is to make sure foundation is applied and blended without flaw. Depending on your skin type, you might want to consider a thicker base

than you would use every day.
Pancake or panstick makeup can
be great for photo shoots, but only
if blended well and applied lightly.
If this type of makeup is applied
too thickly, it may look grainy or
artificial. The color of the foundation should be a perfect match to
the model's neck; you should not
be able to see where the makeup
ends on the jawline.

Learning to contour is one of
the more challenging aspects of
applying professional makeup.
Depending on the shape of your
face, you may need to contour, or
"hollow out," your cheeks. Select
a foundation that is one to two

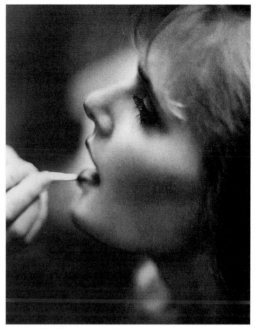

Photo by D. Brian Nelson. © D. Brian Nelson.

shades darker than your skin tone. Suck in your cheeks and feel where
the hollows are under your cheekbones. This area is directly beneath the
cheekbone. Apply the darker shade of foundation in the hollow area in a
upward motion toward your ear. Make sure you blend carefully around
the edges and continue to blend until you see the hollow effect. You
should not be able to tell where you've applied the contour or see any
lines or indication as to where the contour begins and ends.

Another challenge for some beginning models is proper blush application. Look in the mirror and give yourself a big smile. The fullest part of
your cheeks is exactly where your blush should go—not above or below,
but directly on the apple of the cheeks. Using a large brush, apply powder blush in an upward motion, angling toward the ear. Use a sponge or
makeup tissue to blend the blush gently until you have an even, natural-
looking application. Avoid using very dark and drastic colors—the key is
to achieve a healthy glow and emphasize the cheekbones.

Select a neutral, earth–toned eye shadow to contour the eye. With a
small shadow brush, scrape the powdered shadow onto your brush, hold

it away from your face, and blow or shake off the excess powder. This will prevent you from getting dark specks of shadow on your foundation. Apply the shadow along the crease of your eye, starting in the corner and working your way outward. Using a clean brush, blend the shadow until you can no longer see a hard line. You can also use the corner of a clean sponge to blend. Using yet another clean brush, apply a lighter shade of shadow to the bottom, center lid and blend. You can also apply a light shade to the brow bone.

Eyeliner should be applied to the upper lid, beginning at the inner corner and extending across the lid, right at the base of the lashes. Line the lower lid in the same manner, beginning at the inner lid and gently working your way across. Blend eyeliner with a Q-tip or the end of a clean makeup sponge. Make sure the eyeliner is blended well and that there are no smudges around the eye.

After you have completed the foundation, contouring, blush, and eye shadow application, use a translucent, loose powder to set your makeup. The powder needs to be translucent and matte so that it will not interfere with your makeup or change the foundation shade. Apply powder lightly with a large sable brush. It is always advisable to shake off excess powder from the brush so that you can get even coverage without applying too much. Powder should be applied lightly across your entire face, including eyelids. The matte finish of loose powder helps achieve a professional look. You may need to reapply or refresh powder during your shoot; the photographer should direct you to do so if he detects a shine.

Curl your lashes and apply mascara just as you would for everyday wear, but use two coats. Allow a few minutes between applications for the mascara to dry, which will help prevent it from caking.

Always use a lip liner to outline your lips, matching the lip-liner shade with your lipstick. Depending on the look you are trying to achieve, you may want to use lip gloss.

Again, professional makeup technique takes a lot of practice. Be patient, and don't expect perfection overnight.

A New You?

Before you get started on your portfolio, your agent may suggest some things you can do to update your look, like a new hairstyle or different styles of clothing. It is important to trust your agent and the people who are working with you, but you should always go with your instinct and make your own decision. Before I signed with my first agency in New York, I pursued an agency that expressed an interest in signing me, but it was suggested that I accept an appointment with its recommended hairstylist first. It took Pierre two hours to give me a very short and spiky-looking French hairstyle. I went back to the agency expecting to sign

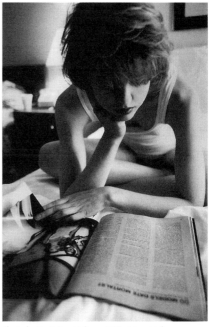

Photo by D. Brian Nelson. © D. Brian Nelson. Model: Leslie Adair.

a contract and was crushed to hear, "We don't like it." I didn't want to go with a short hairstyle but did exactly what the agency suggested in hopes of signing a contract. The clock was ticking, and I wanted to get to work. I didn't want to wait for my hair to grow back.

The agents felt bad; after all, they had suggested I go see Pierre, and they actually told him how they wanted my hair cut. To top it off, I spent more than $100 for the new hairstyle. The agent told me to go home, try to work with it, and see what I could do. I refused to give up because of a bad hair day. While I continued to struggle with a hairstyle I would never have chosen for myself, I finally concluded that in order to impress the agency that had just rejected me, I'd have to find a way, somehow, to feel great about myself–funky hair and all. I spent the next twenty-four hours telling myself how much I loved the new hairstyle. The next morning, I put on my best smile, held my head high, and told myself how much I loved this fun new image. The agent couldn't believe the difference and was thrilled with the results, and I signed my first modeling contract that afternoon. The only real change was my attitude.

Always talk the idea of major appearance changes over with your agent in advance. A major change also means new prints for your portfolio and new composites, so it is not something to do on a whim.

Your image and style are unique and should reflect how you feel and what you believe–don't just copy someone else. A great example of this is model Elle MacPherson. According to a September 21, 1997, article in *Los Angeles Times Magazine,* "Where most fashion models projected haughtiness and aloofness, she was friendly, not distant."

Be yourself, and your image and style will constantly evolve.

Your Portfolio

Your portfolio should ideally contain ten to twelve photographs or tear sheets. The beginning model's portfolio should have:

- One to two headshots, preferably one with a smile and another with a serious expression
- One to two fashion shots
- One to two full–length shots that show your figure

Portfolio books vary in size and style, but the standard book is approximately 9" × 12" with no zipper. Some agencies furnish a portfolio that has the agency's logo on the cover. Depending on the agency, the model may or may not absorb the cost of the book. If the agency does not provide the book and you do not have one, your agent can direct you where to purchase one. You can also refer to Model's Mart (see chapter 20).

The objective you are trying to achieve with your portfolio is to grab someone's attention with your first shot and maintain it throughout the book, leaving the viewer with a strong image at the end. You should strive to show as much versatility as possible.

If at all possible, use more than one photographer to shoot your portfolio. Not only will it give you a more diverse variety of shots, you will gain the experience of working with different professionals. You'll also start to become more comfortable in a photo session.

Do not choose more than one photograph from the same session. You might have several poses in a silky red dress that are fantastic shots—narrow it down to the best one.

Do not overcrowd your portfolio with "good enough" shots. You should feel like all the shots in your book are your best work. I know a famous photographer who tosses all of his photographs that he feels are mediocre and only keeps his outstanding work. He insists this practice maintains his high standards and enables him to keep shooting better images. It is far better to have one fantastic photograph than twelve that are "so-so." If your friend wanted to introduce you to two different people and told you one really great thing about one of them and several "so-so" things about the other, which one would you want to meet first?

In case you thought you'd only have to put together one portfolio book, think again. Agencies work with several books, and once you really get going and have agencies in other parts of the country (or world), you will need several books in those locations (along with stacks of composite cards). These items are all costs incurred by the model. Most duplicate copies of portfolios contain color laser photocopies. Thanks to modern technology, the quality is generally quite good, and duplicates are made at a reduced cost. Even so, the cost to duplicate prints for several books adds up, so be aware.

From the shots contained in your portfolio, you will put together your composite, or "zed," card. This card is your "calling card"; it represents your very best work and contains the images you want to leave with the prospective client. The card is usually comprised of one to four shots from your portfolio, which includes a headshot and a couple of great photos that show different looks. Usually, one of them will show off your figure.

Testings

Most of the major agencies will send their newly signed models for testings so they can start the process of building their portfolio and getting enough great shots to put together a composite. In order to save costs, most agencies will recommend photographers who are willing to do testings. If you are working with a well-known, reputable agency, the photographers have been interviewed, are professional, and can produce the results you need. You might go on as many as ten shoots before having a large enough variety of prints to get started. The testing process is a great way to build your portfolio. The costs you incur should be minimal; they will more than likely include film, developing, and the cost to enlarge the prints you select.

Although the agency supplies a list of photographers who test models, in most cases the model selects the photographer with whom she wants to work. In smaller markets, the model might have to find her own photographers. Some basic things to remember when selecting a photographer who hasn't been screened by your agency are:

- Cost should be kept to a minimum.
- You should not feel pressured in any way to shoot with the photographer.
- You should not be pressured or encouraged to pay a lot of money ($1,000, for example).
- The photographer should not try to get you to shoot your entire portfolio with him.
- The photographer should be more than willing to meet with you and show you his work before you make a decision. Be sure to look at the photographer's contact sheets as well as his book. This will give you better idea as to the quality of the photographer's work.
- You should feel free to take someone along with you to meet the photographer.
- You should feel comfortable with the photographer and the surroundings.

In a testing photo shoot, the model usually supplies props and wardrobe. As a rule, it is the model's responsibility to arrange for the other professionals involved, such as the hairstylist or makeup artist. The exception is when the photographer has something specific in mind that he would like shot for his portfolio.

In most cases, the model should have a basic idea and communicate with the photographer as far as what types of images she wants to create. The photographer may offer suggestions or may want a different type of image for his book. In this instance, the model works with the photographer so that both parties are satisfied with the shoot. The exception is, of course, something the model is not comfortable doing. It doesn't matter if it is a testing or an actual photo shoot for a client; the model should never feel pressured to do anything she doesn't believe in or feel comfortable doing.

It is okay to bring a chaperone to a testing if you have cleared it with your agency and/or the photographer. Most photographers are not offended by this request if they are assured the chaperone will not interfere with their work or yours. However, it is not advisable to bring along a friend if that individual makes you nervous or uncomfortable. This makes your work a lot more difficult and can dull (or end) the creative process. If you are alone, you can remain focused on what you are doing and communicate directly with the people involved on the set.

Model Release

Photographers and clients obtain the right to sell or use pictures of the model by having the model sign a model release. In most instances, the wording of a model release is standard and will contain some of the language given in the following samples. If you are working through an agency, your voucher will probably have a simplified version of a model release (see Example A). Photographers and clients might have their own releases prepared specifically for their purposes.

Model releases are typically signed after the photo session takes place. The request for a model to sign a release is reasonable and customary. Please note that the following sample model releases (Examples B and C) are only guidelines and can be modified to suit the needs of the photographer and/or the model.

~

Example A: Sample Model Release from Agency Voucher

UNIFORM MODEL RELEASE

In consideration of receipt of the fee (inclusive of service fee) negotiated with my manger, I hereby sell, assign, and grant to

_____ (advertising agency or publication) and _____ (client or advertiser) the right and permission to copyright and/or use and/or publish one photograph or likeness of me in which I may be included in whole or in part of composite or reproduction thereof in color or otherwise, in the United States and _____ (other territories) for _____ (usage; for example, print advertising, packaging, point of purchase, etc.) for _____ (product) for _____ months to begin no later than four (4) months from this date.

Accordingly, I release and discharge the companies and persons named above and persons acting for or on behalf of them from any liability by virtue of any blurring, distortion, alteration, optical illusion, or use in composite form that may occur or be produced in the taking of said picture or in any processing thereof through completion of the finished product. All other releases not valid unless countersigned by model's manager.

Client's Representative_____

Model's Signature _____

~

Example B: Model Release

In consideration of my engagement as a model, and for other good and valuable consideration herein acknowledged as received, upon the terms hereinafter stated, I hereby grant _____ (photographer), his/her legal representatives and assigns, those for whom _____ (photographer) is acting, and those acting with his/her authority and permission, the absolute right and permission to copyright and use, reuse and publish, and republish photographic portraits or pictures of me or in which I may be included, in whole or in part, or composite or distorted in character or form, without restriction as to changes or alterations, in conjunction with my own or a fictitious name, or reproductions thereof in color or otherwise made through any media at his/her studios or elsewhere for art, advertising, trade, or any other purpose whatsoever.

I also consent to the use of any printed matter in conjunction therewith.

I hereby waive any right that I may have to inspect or approve the finished product or products or the advertising copy or printed matter that may be used in connection therewith or the use to which it may be applied.

I hereby release, discharge, and agree to save harmless _____ (photographer), his/her legal representatives or assigns, and all persons acting under his/her permission or authority or those for whom he/she is acting, from any liability by virtue of any blurring, distortion, alteration, optical illusion, or use in composite form, whether intentional or otherwise, that may occur or be produced in the taking of said picture or in any subsequent processing thereof, as well as any publication thereof, including without limitation any claims for libel or invasion of privacy.

I hereby warrant that I am of full age and have every right to contract in my own name in the above regard. I state further that I have read the above authorization, release, and agreement prior to its execution and that I am fully familiar with the contents thereof.

Print Name _____

Date _____

Address _____

_____

Signature _____

Witness _____

~

Example C: Model Release for a Minor

In consideration of the engagement as a model of the minor named below, and for other good and valuable consideration herein acknowledged as received, upon the terms hereinafter stated, I hereby grant _____ (photographer), his/her legal representatives and assigns, those for whom _____ (photographer) is acting, and those acting with his/her authority and permission, the absolute right and permission to copyright and use, reuse, publish, and republish photographic portraits or pictures of the minor or in which the minor may be included, in whole or in part, without restriction as to changes or alterations, in conjunction with the minor's own or a fictitious name, or reproductions thereof in color or otherwise, made through any medium at his/her studios or elsewhere, and in any and all media now or hereafter known, for art, advertising, trade, or any other purpose whatsoever. I also consent to the use of any printed matter in conjunction therewith.

I hereby waive any right that the minor or I may have to inspect or approve the finished product or products or the advertising copy or printed matter that may be used in connection therewith or the use to which it may be applied.

I hereby release, discharge, and agree to save harmless _____ (photographer), his/her legal representatives or assigns, and all persons acting under his/her permission or authority or those for whom he/she is acting from any liability by virtue of any blurring distortion, alteration, optical illusion, or use in composite form, whether intentional or otherwise, that may occur or be produced in the taking of said picture or in any subsequent processing thereof, as well as any publication thereof, including without limitation any claims for libel or invasion of privacy.

I hereby warrant that I am of full age and have every right to contract for the minor in the above regard. I state further that I have read the above authorization, release, and agreement prior to its execution and that I am fully familiar with the contents thereof. This release shall be binding upon me and my heirs, legal representatives, and assigns.

Date _____

Name of Minor _____

Name of Parent or Guardian _____

Signature _____

Witness _____

CHAPTER NINE

Congratulations! You Booked the Job!

*"I don't know anything about luck. I've never banked on it, and I'm
afraid of people who do. Luck to me is something else: hard work—
and realizing what is opportunity and what isn't."*

LUCILLE BALL

$\mathcal{M}$ost models remember getting their
first job. What an accomplishment! More than likely, you've been on
several go–sees that led up to this eventful moment. A model's life is
filled with pounding the pavement–often going on as many as ten go-
sees a day. Sometimes you'll simply be meeting professionals to introduce yourself as a new model. At castings, you will be competing for a
specific job.

You will more than likely meet decision makers–those in charge of
choosing the model(s)–at castings. At go–sees, you could meet a variety
of professionals, from the decision makers on down. Magazine editors,
advertising agents, photographers, and catalog editors will look through
your book, shake your hand, and hopefully keep your composite card.

Sometimes you'll go on a callback, visiting the same client for a second time in hopes of landing the booking. This usually means they've

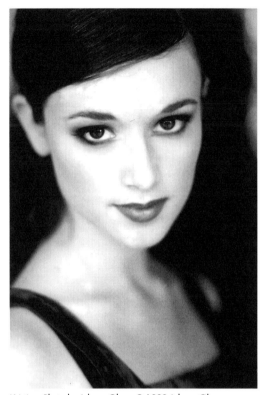

Kristina. Photo by Johnny Olsen. © 1999 Johnny Olsen Photography.

narrowed down their search, and you are among the chosen few who will compete for the booking.

Your first booking could take as little as one hour or as long as a full day. Every job is different; the most important thing to remember is to relax. With every booking you get as a model, your confidence and ability will grow.

Your First Booking

At last . . . you're on your way. Your first booking starts tomorrow. Now what do you do?

Preparation for a job begins the night before. Make sure you completely understand exactly where you are going, how long it takes to get there, and what time you are expected to arrive. Michele August, president of 212 Artist Representatives, Inc., has been everything from model to agent to the owner of a company that represents top fashion photographers. She always encourages her new models to ask questions. "No one is born a model," she advises, "so never be afraid to ask questions. There is no such thing as a stupid question."

The following are some preparation hints and tips on what to expect at a booking:

- The day before the booking, find out if you are required to bring any special items and look through your model's bag to be sure you have everything needed.
- Get plenty of rest. No matter how nervous you might be, go to bed on time.

- Allow plenty of time to get there. You don't want to throw your morning off by struggling to get a cab or speeding to arrive on time.
- You should arrive at your booking with clean hair and a clean face. That means no makeup or hairspray.
- As soon as you arrive, the makeup artist will begin to apply your makeup. This could take up to an hour or more, depending on the booking.
- Next, the hairstylist will style your hair.
- Your wardrobe will be ready, and you will work with the stylist to get ready for the shoot.
- The art director or photographer will communicate their expectations, and you will work with them to produce the desired results.
- Depending on the type of booking, you might be working with other models. If so, be prepared to wait for long periods of time. Be patient and professional.
- Be prepared for anything. Models are often on their feet (in heels) for long periods of time. Your muscles may not be used to stretching and holding a pose. Hang in there.
- Remember, as you become more experienced, bookings will become routine. So relax, be yourself, and try to have fun.

Rates and Scheduling

The agency will set an hourly and day rate for their new models. Once a model starts to work steadily, and as she becomes more experienced and well known, her rates are adjusted. Often models have to travel to locations outside the city and, depending on the terms negotiated by the agent in the booking, are paid for travel time. The payment is not the model's full hourly rate, but generally a flat fee on top of travel expenses. Again, this isn't always the case; these details are determined when the booking is negotiated.

Rates vary by the type of booking. Catalog work pays very well, as does advertising. Although editorial work and magazine covers get you noticed, they do not pay much; fees vary, depending on what is agreed upon by the agent and the editor. Interestingly enough, models who

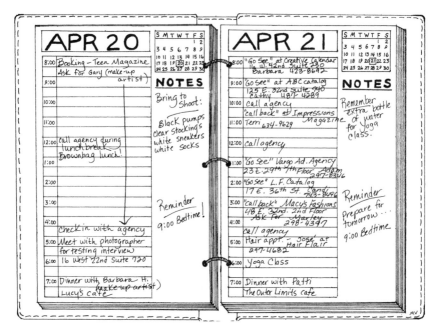

Sketch by Maria Vasseur.

pose in revealing lingerie, bras, underwear, etc., are typically paid double their normal rate. If the undergarments are less revealing, the model will receive one and a half times her hourly rate. If a model decides to do a booking in a garment that is so sheer you can see through the fabric, or in something that is either full or partially nude, the model is paid triple her hourly rate. (This type of modeling refers to fashion only, not spreads in men's magazines.)

Bonus payments or additional fees for exclusive rights to prints are negotiated by the agent and compensate the model for loss of other re-lated work. This fee is in addition to the model's rate and is usually paid upon publication. The amount of these additional fees depends on how the model's image will be used and how often it will appear. The terms may specify anywhere from a three- to twelve-month usage. The client may also opt to pay a "buyout" fee, which will allow for unlimited usage of the image.

Fashion shows generally pay regular hourly or daily rates, depending on the type of show. Less-known or less-publicized shows may command a lower fee. Promotional modeling typically pays less than an hourly rate, often as low as $100 to $300 per day. If the model is booked to show items in stores, the rate could be less than $100 per day.

If a model is fortunate enough to appear in a television commercial, residual payments are paid to the model each time the commercial is aired.

In most of the larger, well-known agencies, the model is paid weekly or every two weeks, even if the client has not yet paid the agency. In some smaller agencies and markets, the payment may not be issued until the agency has been paid. Be sure you have an understanding as to how the payment process works before you sign with an agency, so that there will be no surprises.

If the model knows in advance of a specific period of time in which she does not want to work, she will "book out" for that block of time. This is information to be given to the agent so that nothing will be booked for that period.

Booking Form

Before a model goes out on her first assignment, she will be trained by her agency on how to organize her bookings to make sure she has all the correct information regarding the job and what will be involved. She will also receive vouchers from the agency to use after the job has been completed. These tasks are simple, but extremely important, as they are the tools the model uses to keep her records in order. It is the model's responsibility to make sure there are no misunderstandings about what is needed for a booking and that the client has the proper paperwork needed to pay the agency for her services.

When a booking is made, a model may be responsible for devising her own system to keep track of her assignments. Some agencies offer forms in order to keep track of this information. If you are responsible for devising your own organizational system, the information you need to know for every job is as follows:

- Job date. Make a habit of writing down the day of the week and the date of the booking.

- Time you need to be there. Plan to arrive fifteen minutes early.
- Location. Get exact directions, particularly if you are going to an area with which you are not familiar.
- Fitting date and time.
- Location for fitting. Get directions.
- Duration of the assignment.
- Client.
- Contact name. Who do you ask for when you arrive at the job site?
- Type of product or line of clothing.
- Type of assignment. Is it print work, a fashion show, showroom modeling?
- What you are expected to bring.
- Makeup. Will there be a makeup artist, or should you be prepared to do your own makeup? If you are responsible for makeup, are specific instructions needed? You will need to find out what the client expects (glamorous, natural looking, etc.).
- Hair. Will there be a hair professional on the assignment? If not, find out what the client's expectations are so that you will be prepared. Make sure you allow extra time in advance of the booking to do your makeup and hair if these professionals will not be on the set.

More about Bookings

Some bookings are made several months in advance, particularly if they require travel and the job lasts several days. Other bookings are scheduled at a few days' notice or even at the last minute, only hours before the model is needed. Anything in between is normal, as there is no set standard in this business. Flexibility is a must, changes are frequent, and models need to be able to live with the uncertainty of when they will work again.

Often a model is booked for an assignment for a specified amount of time. If the model does not work the entire agreed-upon length of time, the client must pay her for the time agreed upon, not the time she actually worked.

A definite booking is set when the client selects the model for a job, but sometimes the client is unable to make a decision and will make a tentative booking. This is also referred to as a "hold" or "option" on the model. This essentially means that the client is tentatively reserving the model for a certain time and date. But what happens if another client requests a hold on the model for that same date? That client becomes "second in line" for the model, and the booking is referred to as a "secondary" booking. However, if the second client requests a definite booking, the agent will contact the first client that made the tentative booking and present the option to confirm the booking or release the model to the second (definite) booking. Tentative bookings may be canceled, but if a client cancels a definite booking, the client will be responsible for paying a cancellation fee.

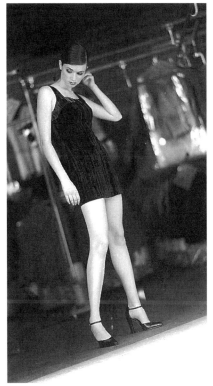

Kristina. Photo by Johnny Olsen. © 1999 Johnny Olsen Photography.

Occasionally, a client isn't certain about a model, or perhaps the details of the advertising campaign are not complete. The model is sometimes hired as a "test" to see if she has the right image to represent the product. The model is typically paid half of her fee for this type of booking, and the rights to the prints are not released. Advertising companies pay huge sums of money for exclusive contracts with models, so hiring a test model is a small investment compared to the extent of work that goes into perfecting the campaign.

Voucher Forms

Voucher forms are used every time a model completes a job. These forms are supplied by the agency and are specific to the agency's billing requirements. Vouchers sometimes come in coupon–type booklets with multiple copies for the client, agency, and model. It is your responsibility to accurately complete the information on the form, because you will not get paid if the form is missing or incorrect. The voucher provides the agency with the necessary billing information and enables it to keep track of the amount owed by the client and the amount due to the model, which will be entered on her ledger sheet.

Included on the voucher is a "model's release." This is usually located at the bottom of the voucher and states that the model releases the rights and grants to the client her permission to copyright, use, and/or publish the photographs from the session. The voucher can waive the model's right to see the prints before publication. The release is not valid until payment is rendered since the model is essentially "selling" the right to use her image in print. The information to be filled out by the model includes:

- Name and address of client.
- Invoice number. (The agency will specify if you are to comply with a billing/tracking numbering system.)
- Product.
- Studio.
- Model's name.
- Model's billing rate.
- Fitting date (time started through time ended) and amount to be charged for fitting (rate multiplied by number of hours).
- Booking date (time started through time ended) and amount to be charged for booking (rate multiplied by number of hours).
- Additional amount charged for booking (negotiated separately).
- Agent's commission (usually 20 percent).
- Additional expenses (as previously agreed upon with client).
- Total amount due.

Be sure you turn in the voucher as soon as possible; if you are late, it could delay the entire billing/payment process. Some agencies charge models a fee for late or delinquent vouchers.

Things You Will Need

Models carry around a lot of items, including things you might not even think you'd need. You must be well organized and prepared for anything that might happen. You never know when you'll have to sew on a button or need an extra pair of stockings. Most agencies will advise you to put together a traveling bag to take on assignments. You can purchase travel-size toiletries to save space in your bag. Here are some suggestions as to what you should have on hand:

- Date/appointment book, calendar
- Pen
- Personal phone/address book
- Money (including change)
- Portfolio
- Vouchers
- Antiperspirant
- Feminine protection
- Extra pair of panty hose (nude)
- Extra underclothing (black, white, flesh color)
- Robe
- Shoes or slippers
- Hairbrush
- Comb
- Curling iron
- Hair drier
- Hair mousse
- Hair pins
- Hairspray
- Hot rollers
- Makeup kit
- Cosmetic brushes
- Makeup remover (or cleanser)
- Mirror
- Moisturizer

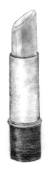

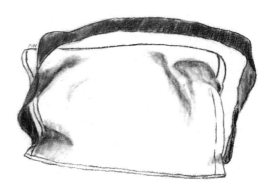

Sketches by Maria Vasseur.

- Sunblock, cream or spray
- Nail file
- Nail polish, clear
- Nail polish, neutral color
- Razor
- Tweezers
- Q-tips (or cotton swabs)
- Tissues
- Safety pins
- Sewing kit
- Protein/nutritional snack bar
- Water bottle

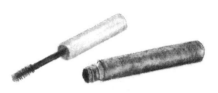

Sketch by Maria Vasseur.

Wardrobe

Additionally, professional models must invest in their wardrobe. Advertisers will typically supply the clothing; however, you need to have some stylish clothes of your own, and, most importantly, you should always have appropriate shoes to complement your outfits. Sometimes, even on big assignments, designers supply the clothes and not the shoes—so you need to be prepared.

Professionalism

There is so much more to modeling than merely sitting in front of the camera and looking pretty. Anyone who thinks that's all there is to it has absolutely no clue as to what professionals go through to get the amazing prints that drive the advertising and fashion world forward. A professional model must develop her own style, know how to apply makeup like a professional, be relaxed and outgoing, and know how to portray different moods for the camera. A professional model must be dedicated, energetic, and very organized.

Some models work for a short period of time, and others manage to turn their work into a long-lasting career. If you want to be the best you can be and really get the most out of your career as a model, consider the following:

- Respect everyone you work with, from the makeup artists to the messengers.
- Do not misrepresent yourself to or withhold pertinent information from your agent, client, or any other professionals with which you interact.
- Maintain your health and be mindful of all factors that reflect your well-being, from watching your diet to getting enough sleep.
- Present yourself in a model-perfect way, well-groomed from head to toe. You should maintain a good manicure, keep your hair trimmed and clean, and maintain good health and hygiene.
- Stay organized so that you will always know where you are going, when you need to be there, and have everything you need to do your best.
- Be on time for your appointments. If you have to miss an appointment, or if something unavoidable prohibits you from keeping your schedule, let the appropriate parties know as soon as possible.
- Have a great attitude; be flexible and upbeat.
- Listen and take direction without demands or complaints. Don't be afraid to ask questions if you don't understand.
- Take care of the client's property. Hang clothes after you have worn them and protect them from damage or stains. If you are modeling a white pullover top, for instance, try to protect the garment from makeup stains.
- Remember that the boss is always right, and in the modeling world, the client is the boss. Never argue with the client.
- Be flexible. If a shoot was scheduled to last two hours but ends up taking four, don't throw a fit or become anxious. Flow with the creative process.
- Take a look at the big picture. In other words, understand and appreciate what the other professionals, from the makeup artist to the photographer's assistant, are doing to create the work at hand.
- Give 100 percent, no matter what.

Keeping Your Balance

Consider yourself truly blessed: You are doing something you love–something that gives you fulfillment! If modeling is the career you want to pursue, maintain your goals and optimism and accept yourself and everything in your life as an opportunity for growth and learning. Be grateful and value all that you have, and don't hesitate to let others know you appreciate them and their efforts on your behalf.

CHAPTER TEN

Avoiding the Dark Side of the Business

"If you have made mistakes, even serious ones, there is always another chance for you. What we call failure is not the falling down, but the staying down."

MARY PICKFORD

*U*nfortunately, there are numerous scoundrels masquerading as agents and photographers. These individuals are basically out to take your money and rob you of your dream. A significant number of scam artists target this profession, and prospective models are vulnerable if they are unaware or naïve. Most of these criminals present themselves as legitimate and lead you to believe that they know what they are doing. They might have a nice office space or run an appealing advertisement in the newspaper. Modeling photos often grace their walls or are presented in books displayed in their offices. So what? The best way to protect yourself from scams or disreputable business practices is to arm yourself with knowledge. Knowledge, coupled with learning to pay attention to your instincts, is the best defense you can have.

Listen to Your Instincts

I've decided to share this personal story with you for two reasons: First, it is a great example of how easily your instincts can be clouded by your dreams; second, it stresses the importance of knowing something about how the business works before you set off to pursue a modeling career. When I first moved to New York, I responded to an advertisement in one of the local trade papers. Although I had received a letter of interest from Ford, I had to wait several months before I could get in to see them. With limited savings, I was anxious to get started and very hungry for an opportunity. Besides, there was no guarantee I would be accepted by Ford.

I had never heard of the agency that had placed the ad, but I can tell you the ad was alluring. I needed money and wanted more than anything to earn it as a model. Thus, I closed my eyes to almost all of the warning signs. When I arrived for my first interview, I noted that the office didn't look like a real modeling agency. There was no receptionist or booker in the office. The phones were not ringing. There were a few chairs in the small waiting room, which were filled with prospective models. There were no photographs of working models on the wall and no agency head books on the tables. But somehow, it was easy to justify this scene. I convinced myself that this was, after all, a new agency. Besides, I was new, so what did I know?

I met and interviewed with a tall, thin, and somewhat nervous man in his fifties. He immediately expressed interest in representing me, pointing out how much he liked my full lips and facial features. He told me I had a very sensual look. When I showed him my portfolio, he seemed interested, pointing out the shots he liked best. I was encouraged when he asked if I would be willing to travel internationally doing fur shows. He claimed most of his clients were based in Singapore, China, and Brazil. He asked me to demonstrate my runway skills, so I walked back and forth in his office. He seemed impressed and encouraged me, saying that I would be perfect for the fur shows. He whipped out a contract and invited me to look it over. It seemed legitimate and generous. My obligation would be a three-month tour at a salary of $1,500 per week, with a signing bonus of $30,000. I was informed that the agency planned to narrow the search to three models and would call me in a few days to let me know where I stood.

Two days later, I was called back for a second interview. Although I was excited about this opportunity, I had more than the normal case of butterflies when I arrived at the agency. For some unexplained reason, I was actually afraid. I told myself that I had spent an entire year preparing for this opportunity. I had fostered such a burning desire to succeed, I talked myself right out of this instinctual warning.

The "agent" told me they'd offered the fur contract to another

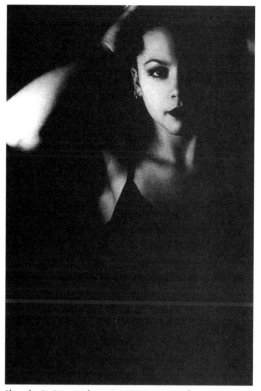

Photo by D. Brian Nelson. © 1999 D. Brian Nelson.

model, but he had something else in mind for me—something better. He needed a model for a new foreign cologne campaign, which he referred to as *Allure*. The *Allure* model would be used in advertisements and would travel on a promotional tour to various countries as a spokesmodel. He showed me a contract that offered the same $1,500 salary per week, all expenses paid, and this time, a signing bonus of $50,000.

I had been in New York for a few months, had gone through most of my savings, and was starting to struggle to make ends meet. This contract seemed too good to be true; I couldn't get the $50,000 bonus out of my mind. I almost had myself convinced that this opportunity was legitimate. Almost.

The next big warning sign slapped me back to reality. The agent asked if I was opposed to posing nude, quickly explaining that the cologne ad was sensual but tastefully done and that it would appear in various foreign magazines. The model would then be required to go on the promotional tour. I couldn't imagine doing a nude ad for cologne; I instantly thought of what my family would think. For some models, this would have been enough to walk out, but I wasn't quite ready to let the $50,000 go.

I explained that I wouldn't be comfortable doing an ad if I had to be *completely* nude, but maybe I would consider partial nudity. I was surprised when he accepted my terms without further discussion. Next, he asked if I had family or a boyfriend that would be at home worrying about me, or if I would request a chaperone on the tour. He strongly suggested that I travel alone, arguing that relatives or friends would only serve to interfere with my career and distract me. Besides, the schedule did not allow for a lot of free time, so everyone would be miserable.

At that moment, I knew without a doubt that this was not only a scam but could potentially be dangerous. This stranger could ship me off to who knows where, and I might not be able to make it back home. I was frightened but pretended to go along with the rest of the interview. I knew that when I walked out of that office, I would never come back. My instincts screamed *danger*, and I couldn't wait to get out of there.

The next day, I called the Better Business Bureau and local authorities, and I was told that this agent would be investigated. I never went back to the agency nor returned his phone calls. I did, however, call the agent's office a few weeks later out of curiosity. The phone had been disconnected. To this day, I don't know the full extent of what this man was up to. I was never asked for money in advance, but the entire experience was creepy and filled me with caution. I was blinded by my dreams. I felt foolish but considered myself lucky that I had the sense to get out of there before any real harm was done.

Advertisements

Be careful if you decide to answer an ad from newspapers or trade papers. Some agency representatives or other presumed professionals advertise for models and offer to conduct interviews at a hotel or apartment. Agencies, school representatives, or photographers rarely conduct interviews at hotels. A convention setting is an exception, but all interviews are conducted in a professional manner and held in public areas.

Beware of an agent who requests an interview after normal working hours or outside of the office. Several years ago, there was a young model who had responded to a classified ad in one of New York's local newspapers. She agreed to meet a modeling agent at a hotel. The agent claimed he was starting up a new agency and his offices were not yet established. But in the meantime, he claimed, he was looking for new models to represent. After the agent greeted her in the lobby, he suggested they go to the room, where he had established his temporary office. The agent claimed the room was only one floor up and suggested they take the stairs. In the stairwell, the model was abducted. This young woman escaped with her life but suffered enough trauma to ruin the pursuit of her dreams.

Beware of ads that indicate "no fee." If it's a scam, at some point you'll be asked to pay money. Legitimate agencies take their commissions from modeling fees earned. (For more information regarding fees and expenses, see chapter 9.)

You might also run across ads for "real–people" types or "kids." These folks ask for all ages, shapes, and sizes. Sometimes these jobs involve the sale of a product and are not real modeling opportunities. You can certainly check them out, but keep both eyes open and leave your checkbook at home.

As a general rule, avoid responding to ads in the "Help Wanted" section of newspapers or local magazines. Most of the time, these ads read something like: "Model Wanted, No Experience Necessary." Some agencies place ads in the classifieds only to get individuals to buy hundreds of dollars' worth of publicity photographs with no intention of getting them work. Parents are ideal targets for such scams. They are told that their child is very special, talented, or beautiful, and if they pay for the photographs, their baby will get commercials or ad campaigns and earn a lot of money. Thrilled at the prospect of having Junior be the next Gerber baby, Mom or Dad plop down the credit card and pay for expensive photographs, but Junior never appears in print.

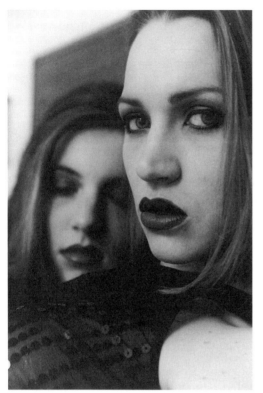

Photo by Stephen Clark. Hotel New York. © 1999 Stephen Clark. Models: Ana and Jes. Makeup: Angela Gallagher.

High Salaries

Unless you know a little bit about this business, you'll probably fall for a line like, "You'll start making a lot of money right away." Any reputable agent will tell you that while it is possible to earn a lot of money in this business, a very small percentage earn tremendous salaries, and rarely immediately. In most cases, models in the high-income bracket have worked at their profession for a long time. It generally takes time for any model to become established enough to start earning a living. In fact, if your agent has advanced you funds for testings, photographs, composite cards, travel, and living expenses, it could take several months of steady work just to reimburse your agency. It takes time to earn tear sheets, build a portfolio, and establish clients. On top of that, there is absolutely no guarantee that you'll work at all. An agency agrees to represent you because its agents believe that you are marketable, so listen to what the company or agency promises and compare it with what you learn about the business. If someone tells you you're going to make a lot of money right away, don't believe it for a minute.

Flexible Schedules

Watch out for agencies that claim their models can work full- or part-time. The fact is, you work when there are jobs. You do go-sees, meet with clients, and compete for jobs when they hold casting calls. There's no room for setting your own schedule. You have to work when they're ready to shoot, not when you can fit it in. And, if you can't make it when they are ready to shoot, there are a few hundred other models that will be more than happy to take your place. One exception to this is if you are in school and do not want modeling to interfere with your education. Then you may start out by working during spring or fall breaks or in the summer.

Modeling Scouts

Most top modeling agencies rely on scouts to recruit new models. Scouts approach potential models on the street, in the store, at the airport, etc. It's certainly possible to run into a scout, agent, booker, photographer, or model manager in any public place. Nevertheless, be wary. If you are ever approached by someone representing himself as a professional, ask for his business number or take his card. Do not ever give him your home phone number or address. Check out strangers before you decide to meet with them to make sure they are legitimate. If you haven't heard of the agency or company with which they are affiliated, check it out. If a scout or agency representative is interested in you, and if he is legitimate, he won't hesitate giving you his business card.

Some modeling scouts work for "agencies" whose sole interest is taking your money. Kenneth Bredemeier, in an April 1999 article for the *Washington Post*, investigated an agency in Fredricksburg, Virginia, and reported that some talent scouts were told by their trainers, "We want you to talk to ten people an hour... I don't care what these people look like, get people in here. Talk to anybody and everybody as long as they're not repulsive to you, as long as they don't turn your stomach." The Federal Trade Commission has since filed suit against three northern Virginia modeling firms, accusing them of engaging in a "fraudulent scheme to lure consumers into signing expensive training contracts without much hope that they would get significant modeling work."

If a modeling scout or agent asks that you pay them, be careful. Know that agencies make money from the fees they charge clients. Most agencies earn their money by taking 20 percent from the client and 20 percent from the model's earnings. The modeling scout is paid by the agency, not the model.

Examining Your Potential

One sure sign you've walked into an agency that's not legitimate is when you hear agents telling nearly everyone who walks in the door that they have what it takes to be a model. Sit down and take a good look at yourself–be honest as you examine your potential for becoming a model. If an agency has offered you representation, ask yourself why. Do you believe the company plans to make money from the clients who hire you, or does it look like it plans to make money from you? Take a look around the waiting room and see what types of models the agency represents. Does it accept anyone and everyone, whether or not they seem to have a chance to succeed?

Investigating an Agency

When it comes to unfamiliar agencies, particularly those in smaller markets, don't be afraid to play detective. Check out all claims made in agency advertisements, sales presentations, and literature. If an agency claims to have launched the careers of famous models, contact other modeling agencies and ask if this is true. It is fairly easy to find out about famous models and discover how they got started. Most agencies and people in this business are very up–front and will give you a straight answer. Don't be afraid to ask for the names and phone numbers of models who work through the agency and follow up with telephone calls to those individuals. You can also ask what clients the agency serves, then call the clients and find out if they utilize the agency you are investigating. If an agency is required by your state to be licensed or bonded as an employment agency, find out if the agency has done so.

Use the Internet to investigate agencies. With more and more people logging onto newsgroups and posting information about their experiences, it will become more difficult for an agency to hide its shenanigans from the public. One great Web site that has a forum on which to post information about scams is *http://modelnews.com*. This site has a "scam watch" category, so if you are unsure of an agency, you can go to this site for help. Do an Internet search—there are many more Web sites like this one.

Money in Advance

Some agencies ask for a lot of money up front, first telling models everything they want to hear—how exquisite they look, how marketable they are, and how much money they can earn. Of course, then the model is asked to immediately invest in an expensive portfolio. While it is true that some legitimate agencies will require you to pay for testings, the cost should be minimal. Depending on your potential and your financial circumstances, some agencies might cover the cost of testings. But if an agency requests that you pay $1,000 or more for a portfolio and use its photographer(s), look out! As previously discussed, most reputable agencies will offer a list of recommended testing photographers, leaving it up to you to decide with whom you want to test. And, the fees should be very reasonable ($25 to $300).

Unprofessional Behavior

Maybe you think it's silly to write about the unprofessional behavior of an agent or photographer who asks a model to remove her clothing. Although it may sound ridiculous, it happens, and all too often, to those who say they'd never do it. I've known models who were lured into situations where they were asked to do something they did not want to do. Some models are so eager to start modeling, or to please the photographer or client, they compromise. This is particularly true with young models who want to present themselves as mature. Given the wrong circumstances and a disreputable professional, before they can say "cheese" they're standing in front of the camera naked.

I knew a New York model who was just getting started and ended up in this type of situation. She returned from a shoot to the apartment building we shared, and I found her up on the rooftop lounge in tears. She couldn't believe that she'd posed without her clothing. She told me how she met a photographer on the subway who offered to test her for the cost of film. She visited his studio in advance and everything seemed okay, so she scheduled the shoot. She brought along several outfits but only made it through two changes. The photographer was very persuasive and made her feel that in order to be a professional, she should be open-minded. She said the experience felt surreal, like everything was moving in slow motion. She didn't know how to say no, and before she knew it, she was posing nude. She felt violated, disappointed in herself, and in shock.

A client or reputable photographer will *never* try to get you to remove your clothing. While lingerie modeling and glamour modeling, or posing nude, are certainly legitimate types of modeling, it is absolutely your choice. Professionals in the industry will respect your choice without reservation. Nudity is something you should feel completely comfortable about. At one time, a model was branded for posing in the buff, but now it is certainly acceptable. In fact, most models in the business today are very comfortable with their bodies, so you see nudity or partial nudity in advertisements and in fashion editorials.

If you are ever presented with an option for work involving nudity or partial nudity, you should have plenty of time to think about the proposed shoot. Your agent or representative should give you all the details, and you should make your own decision without the influence of others. A photo shoot involving nudity should be shot in a professional setting, and you should feel comfortable about it from start to finish. Nothing should ever be "sprung" on you, and you should never feel pressure to do anything that makes you feel uncomfortable

Substance Abuse

What do you do if a photographer or agent offers you a drink or drugs to "settle your nerves"? Plain and simple: Walk out! No questions need be asked, and no discussion is necessary. Just get the heck out of there! This is totally unacceptable and is as far from professional as you can get. It stands to reason that the modeling profession experiences its share of substance abuse; after all, it's a youth-driven, high-pressure, rejection-filled, and often lonely profession, and models can make a heck of a lot of money and find their new wealth hard to handle. It is easily understood how a young model, with no solid home support, thrown into this very "adult" world of fashion, can turn to drugs. If you are serious about achieving success as a model, however, stay away from drugs.

Contracts

Never allow yourself to be pressured into anything–especially when it comes to signing a contract or agreement. Fraudulent agencies or schools will try to get you to sign a contract or document before you walk out of their offices. They do not want you to have time to think about it, and they really know how to put pressure on you. Whatever you do, don't sign or agree to anything until you've thoroughly read it over, thought it over, and discussed it with someone who understands contracts. If an agency is legitimate and interested in you, this request will not be a problem. Your right to request time to think about signing something as serious as a contract is totally reasonable. If you are dealing with a true professional, your request will not be denied.

Conventions

Modeling conventions can be a great opportunity to learn more about the industry, meet professionals, attend workshops, and, most importantly, meet with representatives from some of the top agencies in the country. Conventions can also be a complete rip-off! The two main questions you should ask before you consider attending a convention is: (1) what agencies are represented, and (2) how much does it cost?

When I first started to research this book, a model sent me an e-mail indicating that she was almost taken in by a company that sponsored conventions. The advertisement she had responded to reported that a certain famous model was discovered through this company's convention and indicated that "You can, too." The young girl decided to check it out and attended a couple of the classes. Auditions were held for prospective models who wanted to attend the convention. The model was told she "made it" through the first audition process and could attend. Then her parents were given a pamphlet that indicated the $4,000 cost for attending the convention. After they refused to pay that much money, this organization called again to see if they would be interested in a private interview with an agent at a cost of $30. The model and her parents decided that this operation was a rip–off, and they were absolutely right. No modeling school or model management company should charge you money for the opportunity to meet with an agent. Sure, conventions cost money, but worthwhile conventions charge reasonable fees, certainly not $4,000.

There are some very reputable, sincere people who host conventions across the country. These conventions are a lot of fun, very informative, and give the model an opportunity to meet with quite a few major agency representatives at a reasonable cost. (For further information, see chapter 18.)

Schools

Watch out for agencies that claim you'll only get work after you pay for training. Reputable agencies will generally groom models and let them learn their trade as they work. Modeling, in general, does not require formal training.

Some modeling schools have served to help models gain poise, confidence, and exposure to agencies, and some girls find modeling schools valuable for the grooming advice alone. Investigate modeling schools just like you'd investigate an agency. Some states require that a school or agency be licensed or bonded, so find out if the school you are interested in meets those requirements. While you are at it, verify that its bond/ license is current.

Do not sign for or agree to modeling classes before you are eligible to work. A legitimate agency will groom you and offer training but won't charge you for classes. There is an exception, however. There are some schools that also serve as modeling agencies. These modeling schools charge for classes, acting as separate entities within the agency. A good example of a legitimate school is the Nancy Bounds Studio, located in

Omaha, Nebraska. This is a very successful school, one that is well respected in the industry by some of the top agencies. This school has produced several working professional models.

Federal Trade Commission

If you have paid money to a modeling agency and believe you have been taken advantage of, you should request a refund. If you are not satisfied, register a complaint with your local consumer protection agency, Better Business Bureau, and state Attorney General's office. Also, contact the advertising manager of the newspaper that ran the ad you answered. For ethical and practical reasons, the advertising manager may be interested to learn about any problems you have had with the offending advertiser.

You can also write to: Correspondence Branch, Federal Trade Commission (FTC), Washington, DC 20580 to request the free pamphlet, *Facts for Consumers: Modeling Agency Scams*. This pamphlet provides general information as well as a listing of FTC offices in cities throughout the United States. Although the FTC cannot represent you directly in a dispute with a company, the commission can take action if it finds evidence of a pattern of deceptive or unfair practices. The FTC regularly compiles reports on such companies. You can also file a complaint with the FTC by contacting the Consumer Response Center at (202) 382–4357 or (202) 326–2502. The Bureau of Consumer Protection Offices of Consumer and Business Education can be reached by calling (202) 326–3650. To file a complaint or obtain more information via the Internet, go to the FTC's Web site, *www.ftc.gov*. The FTC also has offices in Atlanta, Boston, Chicago, Cleveland, Dallas, Denver, Los Angeles, New York, San Francisco, and Seattle.

CHAPTER ELEVEN

Travel and Relocation

"When you get into a tight place and it seems you can't go on, hold on, for that's just the place and the time that the tide will turn."
HARRIET BEECHER STOWE

*M*ost models travel extensively and work all over the world, so they must be flexible and ready to travel at the drop of a hat. The heartbeat of the industry is in New York City, so this chapter is devoted to temporary housing and relocation in New York, along with international travel tips. Although most of the major international modeling markets are covered in the next chapter, this chapter offers basic information on international travel.

Relocating to New York

Manhattan is, by far, the largest and most challenging market you'll find when it comes to modeling. It can certainly be intimidating to think about moving to this great city if you are from a small town. If you are presented with a chance to move to New York, hopefully you'll be working with an agency that will help you get established by placing you in a

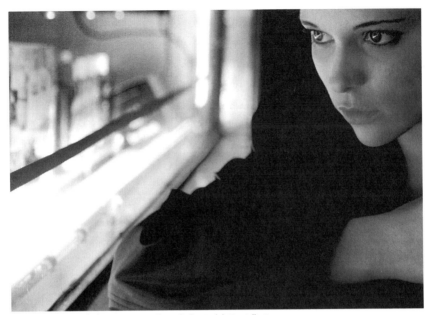

Photo by Stephen Clark. © 1999 Stephen Clark. Model: Danielle Peterson.

models' apartment and helping you get acclimated to the city. If that's the case, your relocation needs will basically be taken care of by the agency with the stipulation that you will reimburse the agency for any or all expenses incurred as you are established.

Although agencies often help a new model find housing, they generally don't serve as a "babysitting service" (as one agent put it). They will help give directions, advise on professionals such as makeup artists, hairstylists, and other professionals, but learning to get around is basically up to the model. Like anything else, there are exceptions. Some agencies have been known to have a full-time chaperone for a very young model when a parent or guardian is not able to fulfill that need.

If you decide to move first and then set out to find an agency, you'll be working a lot harder to make this transition. So where do you start?

Learning about New York

The one thing that helped me out more than anything when I moved from a small town in West Virginia to New York City was reading everything I could get my hands on. By the time I made my first trip, I felt like I knew the city. I had studied maps, landmarks, and the city's history. I found out everything I could about transportation and knew about job availability at temporary agencies. I had a hotel reservation in a safe part of the city and several leads on permanent housing. It was a very smooth transition for me, but only because I took the time and effort to thoroughly prepare. Once you get to New York, invest in a good street map and subway map. You can find a copy of the *NYC Taxi and Limousine Drivers Guide* in most drugstores and newsstands in the city, which is a great guide to help you get around.

Hotels

The following hotels represent a variety of price ranges and are geographically close to most of the top modeling agencies:

Beekman
575 Park Avenue
New York, NY 10021
(212) 838-4900

Lombardy
111 East 56th Street
New York, NY 10022
(212) 753-8600

Gramercy Park Hotel*
2 Lexington Avenue
New York, NY 10010
(212) 475-4320

Madison Towers
22 East 38th Street
New York, NY 10016
(212) 685-3700

Loews New York
569 Lexington Avenue
New York, NY 10022
(212) 350-6048

Sherry-Netherland
781 Fifth Avenue
New York, NY 10022
(212) 355-2800

*Probably the closest hotel to most of the agencies, including Elite, Wilhelmina, Gilla Roos, Ikon, Images Management, IMG Models, Maxx Men, Zoli, Generation, and Marilyn, Inc.

Residences

I didn't know anyone when I moved to New York, but I was fortunate to stay at The Parkside Evangeline, a women's residence located in Gramercy Park, a beautiful, exclusive, and safe neighborhood between Park and Third Avenues. The residence building itself is safe, clean, and charming. Rent is paid on a weekly basis at a very reasonable rate and comes with two meals per day.

This residence is run by the Salvation Army and was established to help young women "get a start" in the city. Since it is a women's residence, men are not allowed past the first floor. Most of the rooms have their own bathrooms, and there are common quarters including a lobby area, dining rooms, solarium, sun deck, and a rooftop lounge area. A tremendous added benefit is the opportunity to meet other young ladies pursuing various careers. This residence is geared toward females between the ages of eighteen and thirty-five.

I made lifelong friends while residing at the Parkside. My transition from a small town to a big city was much easier because of the instant friendships I was able to make. The Gramercy Park location is another reason I highly recommend this residence. There is a waiting list, so you might want to inquire well in advance of your departure. The Parkside Evangeline and other residences are listed below. (The ❋ symbol indicates women's residences.)

The Parkside Evangeline Residence ❋
18 Gramercy Park South
New York, NY 10003
(212) 677-6200

Katherine House ❋
118 West 13th Street
New York, NY 10011
(212) 242-6566

The Markle Residence ❋
123 West 13th Street
New York, NY 10011
(212) 242-2400

Carmelite Sisters ❋
249 West 14th Street
New York, NY 10011
(212) 242-8224

Centro Maria Residence ✳
539 West 54th Street
New York, NY 10019
(212) 757-6989

Fashion Institute of Technology
210 West 27th Street
New York, NY 10009
(212) 760-7885

Sacred Heart Residence ✳
43 West 20th Street
New York, NY 10012
(212) 929-5790

Ten-Eyck Troughton Residence ✳
145 East 39th Street
New York, NY 10016
(212) 490-5990

International House *(foreign students)*
500 Riverside Drive
New York, NY 10027
(212) 678-5000

Short-Term Housing
Euro Casa Connection: (212) 243-2471
Maison International: (212) 462-4766
New York Habitat: (212) 255-8018
West Side YMCA: (212) 787-4400

If you are interested in investigating a women's residence as a place from which to get established in the city, check postings at colleges or in the papers. If you end up signing a contract with an agency, they will more than likely help you find a new place to live, possibly in their models' apartments.

International Travel

The first two things you should do if you think you will be traveling internationally is (1) get your passport application under way and (2) find a good travel agent. The best way to find an agent is to ask your agency and other models who they use. Many fashion-industry professionals in New York prefer The Frenchway Travel Agency, at 11 West 25th Street, because it provides the best rates available and caters to fashion-industry professionals who have to deal with quick changes. Several professionals report that they can get last-minute tickets at a good price. You can reach the agency by phone at (212) 243-3500 or by fax at (212) 243-3535.

If you have the opportunity to travel internationally, your agency should help prepare you by providing all the information you will need.

You can also go the extra mile yourself and do research on your own about where you will be traveling. You should try to learn everything you can about your destination before you take off. Take advantage of your local library and travel agency to find out about customs, currency, geography, etc.

It sounds incredibly glamorous and exciting to hop on a jet and fly off to a foreign country to pursue a modeling career, but don't think for a second that it comes without obstacles. Being prepared and knowing what to expect can help you overcome some of those less-glamorous moments. Karim Ramzi, a well-known photographer from Paris, advises, "First of all, do your homework. Know where you are going in Paris and make sure you have a couple of contacts in case of emergency. The biggest problem for most models who arrive in France is the fact that they do not speak French and therefore have trouble with communication." If you know in advance what other models have run up against and what you should expect, you can overcome, or at least be prepared to handle, adverse situations a little easier.

Make sure you have travel insurance, health insurance, and a sufficient amount of money (traveler's checks). You should also have a working understanding of how taxes and work permits are handled in these markets; different countries vary on requirements and regulations. As discussed in previous chapters, many agencies advance fees for housing and other expenses incurred while traveling internationally. All of these details should be understood without question before you leave.

You may find it hard to believe that you would ever be homesick while leading this glamorous life, but when you are swept away from the comfort and familiarity of your friends and family and find yourself in a foreign country with strange food, a different language, and a whole new way of life, you might discover that you desperately miss home. If you think that you might experience homesickness, plan out ways to combat the emotion. You can find a cybercafé in Paris and keep up with your friends and family via e-mail. Get to know other models. Learn about the country. Continuously tell yourself that this assignment is temporary, a great opportunity, and a tremendous investment in your future as a model (or anything else you want to pursue).

Your Passport

If you don't have a valid passport, your agent should provide you with details on how to obtain one. Make sure you apply well in advance of your first international booking, because the process often takes several weeks. However, it is a simple process that requires filling out an application and submitting the following:

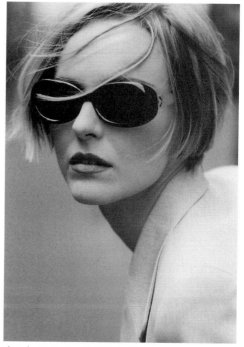

Photo by Karim Ramzi. © Karim Ramzi.

- Proof of citizenship. Acceptable documents include a birth certificate, certificate of citizenship, report of birth abroad, or evidence of citizenship through naturalization of parent(s).
- Proof of identity. A photo identification document, such as a previous U.S. passport or driver's license. If you do not have photo identification, you must appear with an identifying witness who is a U.S. citizen or permanent resident who has known you for at least two years. Your witness must prove his/her identity and complete and sign an affidavit before the acceptance agent.
- Photographs. You must submit two identical, passport–size photographs of yourself, which can be obtained at one of the many places that offer passport photo services.

The passport fee is $45, with an additional charge of $15 for execution of the application. Your passport is valid for ten years. It takes a few weeks to receive a passport in the mail, but expedited service is available for an additional fee of $35. (You may be asked to provide proof of travel for expedited service.) These requests can be processed in three working days after receipt at a passport agency.

Money, Traveler's Checks, and Foreign Currency

One of the most important things you will need when traveling internationally is plenty of money. Your agency should suggest the amount you will need and may be able to advance you some money. It is difficult enough to be in a foreign city and have to find your way around and cope with a different language without having to worry about foreign currency. You don't need to add to that stress by not having enough money to pay for taxis. Make sure you have cash in the currency of the country you are working in before you take off and have an understanding of the exchange rate and terminology. Once you get settled, you can make arrangements to visit a bank and have your traveler's checks or cash converted as needed. Take traveler's checks with you and keep the receipt or numbers of the traveler's checks in a separate location. It is a good idea to purchase a round-trip ticket or have the funds set aside for a return airline ticket.

Keep your most important possessions with you (in your carry-on bag) and not in the luggage you check with the airline. Specifically, you should have your address book, contact names and telephone numbers, portfolio, composites, and passport. It is essential to have the following handy as well:

- Names, addresses, and telephone numbers of your agency contacts
- Hotel/apartment address and phone number
- American Consulate contact information
- Foreign language dictionary

One last word regarding international travel: You need to understand how telephones work in various countries. This might sound ridiculous, but horror stories about models who arrive in Paris and are not able to get the phones to work are common. Find out about purchasing a phone card before you travel or get information about the telephone system of the country you are visiting.

❧

CHAPTER TWELVE

International Modeling

"In the middle of difficulty lies opportunity."
ALBERT EINSTEIN

One of the greatest things about modeling is the opportunity to travel and see the world–if you are ready. If you are under the age of eighteen, it is advisable to travel with a companion; e.g., mother, aunt, sibling, etc. For those who are very young and not ready to be on their own, being in a foreign country can be lonely, intimidating, and overwhelming. You've got to be ready and know what you are getting into in order to survive and be happy working in other countries.

There is plenty of work for beginning models in foreign markets. Depending on your type and marketability, your agent may suggest sending you abroad to work for months at a time. It is common for a new model to start out where she can gain experience and (more importantly) tear sheets before returning to one of the major U.S. markets. There are so many fashion magazines and designers based in Europe, it makes sense that this would be a great place to launch a modeling career.

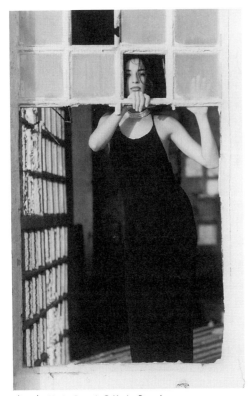

Photo by Karim Ramzi. © Karim Ramzi.

It is advisable to work through an agency in the United States and not set off to international markets on your own. It is also important to stick with your agency and not be lured away while you are working in another country.

This chapter will give you a basic idea of the various types of modeling that can be found in the international markets. I also highly recommend reading *The Modeling Handbook*, by Eve Matheson, for specific information and true stories about international modeling. Eve has traveled all over the word, remains in close contact with agents and models, and offers a wealth of information on what to expect.

Just as people can have different body types from race to race or country to country, you will find that physical requirements for models vary according to venue. If you find that you are generally too short for modeling in New York, for example, you might be able to develop an outstanding career in Asia. Whether you plan to start your career in Milan and then return to the United States or even if you have plans to become a world traveler, you should nevertheless familiarize yourself with the varying standards around the world.

Australia

The basic height requirements for models in this country are 5'8" to 5'10" for women and 5'11" to 6'0" for men. Sydney is mostly known for editorial fashion and advertising and Melbourne is known for catalog. Australia is a fun and interesting place to work and offers a year-round market. Successful models in this market have a casual, neat, and clean look.

England

The types of modeling work available in London are editorial, runway, and advertising. London is known for being one of the tougher markets and typically uses models who have more experience. The foreign agency will help the model obtain a working visa, which usually takes about four weeks. Basic height requirements for London are approximately 5'9" to 6'0" for women and 5'11" to 6'2" for men. Agencies in London expect a high level of professionalism.

The two main airports here are Heathrow and Gatwick. Transportation is fairly reasonable and available–from the "tube" (the subway) to double-decker buses and taxis.

France

The basic height requirement for female models in France is 5'9". The various types of work include editorial, runway, commercial, and catalog. Paris is one of the most exciting cities in the world when it comes to fashion. The beginning model can get off to a great start in Paris and does not need tear sheets in order to do so. You will find a lot of modeling agencies in the "City of Lights," but most prefer to work with an American model through an American agency–it is not advisable to show up there without a home-base or "mother" agency. Although you can find inexpensive housing, Paris is generally an expensive city, so you must have enough money to sustain you for a few months while you get started. Also be prepared to pay very high commission and tax rates (more than 50 percent). August and September are not good months to get settled into the Paris modeling scene–in August, a lot of people take a month-long holiday, and September is booked with fashion shows and the collections.

There are plenty of photographers to test with in Paris. You can find samples of their work in *Le Book* (*www.lebook.com*), which lists photogra-

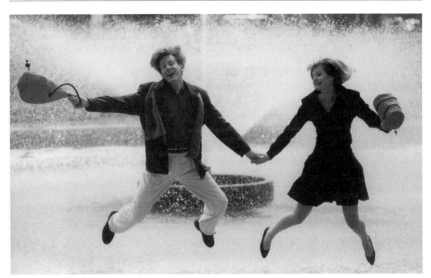

Photo by Karim Ramzi. © Karim Ramzi.

phers, makeup artists, modeling agencies, and magazines. Even if you sign with an agency, you will still need to work on your book. Take advantage of what these professionals have to offer.

The two major airports are Charles de Gaulle and Orly. You can utilize taxis or a bus to get to the city. The subway system is called the Metro, but it is advisable to become more familiar and comfortable with the city before giving it a try.

Germany

Modeling work available in Germany consists mostly of catalog and advertising, with very little editorial and runway work. Female models are generally 5'8" to 6'0" in height; male models are 6'0" or taller.

Hamburg and Munich are the main markets. Since Germany is a major fashion exporter, a model's bread and butter will more than likely be catalog work, so tear sheets earned may not be suitable for use in other countries. Models can earn decent wages and find plenty of work in Germany, but expectations concerning a model's professionalism and ability to follow directions are extremely high. You must be on time and exhibit a very good work ethic in order to be successful here.

Hamburg is a great place for a young model. Most people speak English, and you'll find they are friendly, helpful, and honest. You might be surprised to learn that a lot of German clients like to shoot in America, particularly Miami. Another great thing about Hamburg is that some agencies will place a model in a home with a German family, which offers a little more stability. A model with a strong enough book to impress the German market can start working immediately, but if she needs to do testings and build her portfolio, it could be several weeks before she starts to work. Of course, there are no guarantees–it can often take months to really get started. The airport for Hamburg is Fuhlsbuttel, and from there you can take a taxi or the subway (U–Bahn) into the city. It is recommended that you explore the U–Bahn only after you have been in Hamburg a while.

Munich is the major fashion market in Germany, with "Fashion Week" taking place in March and October. It is more difficult to start out in Munich than Hamburg because of the trend in Munich to work with more experienced models. You must have a good portfolio and composites to work in this Bavarian city, and you must also know how to apply your own makeup like a professional. The airport that services Munich is Flughafen Riem, from which you can utilize bus service, taxis, the train (Hauptbahnhof), or U–Bahn.

Greece

Athens is a good place for new models to get tear sheets since it is a smaller, less competitive market. You don't need a lot of prints in your portfolio to get started here.

Italy

The minimum height requirement for female models in Italy is 5'9". The types of work (predominately in Milan, not Rome) include editorial, advertising, runway, and commercial. There are probably more fashion magazines in Milan than in any other market, which is why you'll find so many models there. Milan is a great place for a beginning model–you don't need tear sheets, and you can build your portfolio quickly. This market is highly competitive, so you should feel very positive about your potential and have a great U.S.–based agent working with you. As in most of the major international cities, you should definitely arrive with enough money to survive for several months. Milan is expensive, and living conditions and models' apartments might not be the greatest. Be sure you have an understanding about your living arrangements before you arrive so that there will be no surprises. One final note: Don't expect to earn and save a lot of money in Milan, even if you are working steadily. Agencies in Milan take about 50 percent of your earnings, which covers taxes and commission. Just remember–you're building a terrific portfolio. The two airports in Milan are Linate and Malpensa, both of which are serviced by taxi and bus service.

Japan

Although the height requirements vary, the standard desired height for models in Japan is 5'7" to 5'9". This market offers mostly catalog and advertising work, and some editorial. The major fashion market in Japan is in Tokyo, which offers editorial work; commercial and catalog work are mainly found in Osaka. Most models who work here are booked for two months at a time. One of the greatest things about the Japanese market is that all of the arrangements are predetermined: Your round–trip airfare and accommodations are advanced, and you will be guaranteed a minimum amount of money whether you are booked or not. In this market, you will be expected to supply accessories, be very professional, and work hard. Most models report having a fun time working in this market–they learn a lot while earning a decent amount of money.

Kristina Proulx, a model with Model Management International (MMI), has had three years' worth of great experience as a model in the Asian market. "Japan is a wonderful place to work," she advises. "The people there are really nice. If you go to Europe, you are left more on your own. In Japan, you have a manager who helps you out, the other models are very supportive, and it isn't as competitive. It's great for young people to go there first, before they go to Europe." Kristina has balanced high school (and now college) with her modeling career, modeling during school breaks and over the summer.

Schedules are very structured in the Asian market. For example, a model could go on as many as ten castings in a day—or work a job and go on castings afterward. Sometimes transportation to castings is provided. There's always someone around who speaks English to help interpret, so communication is generally not a problem.

The two airports that service Japan are New Tokyo International and Haneda. Transportation, from taxis to the subway, is fairly simple and efficient.

Scandinavia

Most assignments in Norway, Sweden, and Denmark are made in advance. Surprisingly enough, exotic, dark-haired models do well in this market.

Spain

In Spain, the height requirement for female models is 5'8". The Spanish market is growing fast and offers the beginning model opportunities in television commercials, as well as editorial, advertising, and catalog work. Spain is a good choice for beginners because of its friendliness, willingness to help, and high-quality editorial work. Better still, the commissions and cost of living in Spain are less than in Paris or Milan.

Switzerland

The available types of work in Switzerland are catalog and commercial print. Zurich is the major fashion market in Switzerland, which is not highly recommended for beginners because clients expect experienced models who already have tear sheets. Models without them are usually sent to Italy to gain experience before working in Zurich. To work in

Switzerland, you must know how to do your own professional makeup, and it is expected that the model supplies the accessories on a shoot. Transportation is simple: There is no underground train or subway; taxis, buses, and trams are the easiest way to get to and from the Zurich airport.

CHAPTER THIRTEEN

Modeling and the Internet

"We all have possibilities we don't know about.
We can do things we don't even dream we can do."
DALE CARNEGIE

*T*here are vast amounts of information about modeling and industry resources available on the Internet, including agency information, interviews with top models, and tips on how to get started. In addition to conventional and well-known agencies offering Web sites, there are companies that directly promote models via the Internet and models who promote themselves in cyberspace. In terms of this industry, use of the Internet is a new frontier and is certainly an exciting way to explore the business of modeling. (To start your own exploration as to what type of information you'll find in cyberspace, there are a wealth of Web sites listed in chapter 20.)

Due to the impact of the Internet, the modeling industry is just beginning to experience changes in the way business is conducted. Composites and model information can be viewed at anytime, day or night, from anywhere in the world, allowing agencies instant access to this information. Models and prospective models can also utilize the Web to find out about agencies, other models, and just about anything else they want to know about the business.

Online Agencies

The number of modeling agencies that have Web sites is growing every day. Some of the well-known agencies, like Ford, Elite, and Wilhelmina, have an Internet presence yet are reluctant to express what they think this technology will do for them in the future. Some of the newer agencies, like Q Model Management Online at *www. qmodels.com,* are more progressive and innovative when it comes to use of Web technology. As a prospective model, you can e-mail your pictures (in JPEG or GIF format), and the company claims you will receive a response within twenty-four hours.

If you decide to send your photographs to a modeling agency via the Internet, make sure you use the same guidelines that you would if you were sending photographs through the mail. Your photographs should be clean, natural shots. Do not send any more than two shots: one that shows your figure and one headshot. Glamorous shots with overdone makeup are not desirable, and professional photographs are not needed. You can have a roll of film developed onto a disk, select two shots, and send them to the agency electronically.

Investigating Scams

In conducting research for this book, I discovered how amazingly easily it was to find out about the reputations of agencies through the Internet. From model newsgroups to some of the Web sites described in chapter 20, you can find out details on how some agencies and schools try to take advantage of models and students. Obviously, the Internet is not the only way to investigate an agency or school, but it is a great place to start.

Forums and Chat Sites

As with any other topic of interest, there are several chat sites and newsgroups available where models, agents, photographers, and other professionals meet online. This is a great place to get to know the busi-ness and the players and is also a forum in which you can ask questions.

Sleazy Sites

Once you start exploring the Internet for modeling–related sites, you will likely run into a few sleazy sites. Unfortunately, some of these sites come up when you search for "models" or "modeling" using search engines like Alta Vista or HotBot. Fortunately, most of the pornographic sites have an advanced warning before you launch into the site, so don't go into shock if you pull some of them up in a search–just leave the site as soon as you are forewarned. Your results will be cleaner if you search under the words "fashion model" instead.

~

A Model's Web Page

A growing number of beginning models are creating their own Web pres-ence. Luria Petrucci is a wonderful example. This young, innovative model thoroughly did her homework before pursuing a modeling career. In her own words, Luria explains why she decided to build her Web site, *http: //luriapetrucci.com:*

> The real strength of the Internet is that it provides a way to reach out and communicate with people who share your goals and interests. When I decided to pursue modeling, going online seemed like a natural step to promote what I was doing and to get feedback and advice from anyone interested enough to give it.
>
> As I learned more about the modeling business, I began to see a major difference between girls who make really good money as models and those girls we affectionately call supermodels. The thing that sets models like Cindy Crawford, Kate Moss, Claudia Schiffer, and newer models like Tyra Banks, Heidi Klum, and Rebecca Romijn-Stamos apart from the thousands of girls whose names we don't know is that they've worked to establish their names as recognizable brands. Cindy Crawford

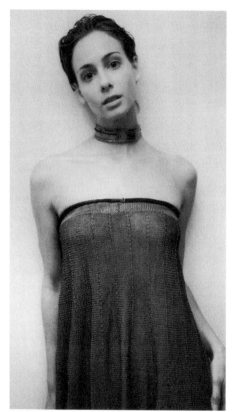

Luria Petrucci. © 1999 LuriaPretrucci.com. Boyer Kloster, Photographer.

is a great example. She's done such a brilliant job of searing her name into the public consciousness that she will be able to sell things just with the value of her name long after her looks fade—if they ever do.

Modeling is all about attracting attention to a particular product. I wanted to prove to myself that I have ability to attract that kind of attention. The response [to my Web site] is beyond anything I could have anticipated. In its first month, *luriapetrucci.com* has had more than 6,000 unique visitors. Since one of the things I wanted to accomplish on the Internet was to demonstrate my ability to sell, I created an e-commerce section for my site to sell posters, prints, and CD-ROMs. The site made a profit in its first month.

I receive hundreds of e-mails filled with the most encouraging and supportive words. Much to my surprise, I have only received one negative message and nothing strange or too outrageous. Everyone has been so polite and helpful. The whole experience has built my confidence and given me courage to really pursue my dream.

As for modeling, everything is happening so fast that I don't know what will be next. I hope to be working in Europe or New York soon. One of the real secrets of success in modeling seems to be having an agent who is completely passionate about your career. I really believe in living with passion, and I look forward to that kind of collaboration.

∼

Cyber Models

Most professionals in this industry insist that a model should have agency representation in order to achieve success. There are so many variables to consider when trying to model without representation, but the most important one is safety. Reputable agencies know their clients and won't put you in any compromising situations. If you are in an uncomfortable situation, you have the agency to act on your behalf, settle disputes, and guide your career. There are instances, however, where models work independently through the Internet. To work independently and promote oneself this way takes an individual with maturity, computer skills, a marketable look, and one who lives in or near a metropolitan area. Internet model promotion is still relatively new, but it seems to be increasing by leaps and bounds.

Working independently requires a lot more networking and marketing on your part. You are responsible for the business details, such as billing the client, promoting yourself, and putting together your composite cards and portfolio. You will need to network with photographers to see if they can use you or help you find clients. It will be up to you to contact and visit companies, advertising agencies, department stores, and so on, and leave your composite with them to try to get work. This is not a conventional way of modeling, so please, be very careful if you decide to model independently.

You can also promote yourself through a model management company or agency that posts models on the Web. For example, America Model Promotions at *http://americamodels.com* will post your modeling portfolio online. You can either send them prints to scan in or e-mail attachments such as JPEG or GIF files. America Models is not an agency or model management company; it merely serves to help you, the model, gain exposure on the Internet. Modeling agencies, photographers, clients, and scouts can contact you directly via e-mail or by telephone–but don't list your home address or telephone number. If you give a telephone number, make sure it is an answering–service number or message machine. Please note that America Models will only accept members who are eighteen years old or older. Since this type of service is new, there has not been enough time to determine the long-term success rate for models who use this or any other Web site for promotion.

Another option is to use bulletin boards or newsgroups to promote yourself. If you have your own Web site, you can post your portfolio and market yourself that way. When you send an e-mail, you can then list the URL (Uniform Resource Locator, or Web site location) in your e-mail "signature." You might be surprised how many people will take a look.

Some additional precautions are necessary if you are an independent model. You should establish a modeling identity (a pseudonym) and get an answering service to take your calls. You should give out your composite card with this "working" name and number represented, not your personal information. When you go out on a job or interview, tell someone where you are going. Check out the location in advance and get a sense as to whether it seems legitimate and safe. Make sure you get all the details first before you agree to do a job. Find out what it pays, the specifics of the job, and what the client's expectations are. Note: There should be a release with all the agreed-upon details waiting for you to sign when you reach a job. Just in case there isn't, take a couple of copies of your own along.

Keep in mind that it will take a while to get started. You may not make money right away, but you will have expenses to cover. More than likely, you will need to have an additional means of support.

As an independent model, you will be responsible for negotiating your fee, so it is up to you to know what agencies charge per hour for various jobs for models of your type in your region. You should charge less than the agency charges since you are not paying commission out of that fee.

Katwoman.com

Cyber model Shannon Marie Codner, whose Web site is *www.katwoman.com*, has been modeling independently via the Internet for more than three years. She was one of the first models to use the Internet and didn't know of any other models at that time who were promoting themselves this way. It took quite a few months to get started, but it paid off. Shannon usually works four days a week, sometimes at more than one booking per day. She has even traveled internationally to work and claims to have had very few negative experiences in her modeling career. One incident, as Shannon explained, was clearly not professional: "I met with a photographer to discuss a potential on–location photo shoot, and he seemed okay. Then, when it came down to us setting up a shoot, he freaked out when I wanted to bring a chaperone with me. He claimed that it would be impossible for me to do that because his photographer's insurance only covered him and a model. Needless to say, I broke off all contact with this guy."

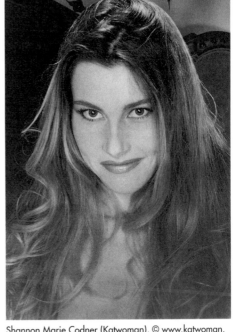

Shannon Marie Codner (Katwoman), © www.katwoman. com. Photo by Dan Peterson.

Shannon also works with stock photography and has some regular clients. Contracts for jobs vary–sometimes she requests a flat fee or claims a percentage when the image sells. She maintains the rights to some of her photos and participates in testings with photographers. She models mostly sportswear, lingerie, fitness gear, and swimwear.

As an independent model, Shannon is responsible for negotiating her fees, which vary depending on the project and what she's modeling. She also utilizes her Web site to sell fashions and other items. Many times, if she's modeling for a specific company, she'll offer to sell the merchandise through her Web site in exchange for a percentage of the sales that are made.

Advice for Cyber Models

- Start with a listing of photographers in your area. Call or stop by their studios and review their work. Arrange for testings.
- Don't pay for prints unless you want something specific with a certain photographer.

- Decide what type of modeling you want to specialize in (swimwear, fashion, lingerie, etc.).
- Check out Geocities or Tripod and get your prints on the Web. Advertise that you need prints for your portfolio.
- When screening clients and/or photographers, ask for their Web site. If they don't have one, ask them to send copies of their work or something about their company to your post office box (not your home address). Offer to return their prints after you've had a chance to review them. Ask for contact information for other models they have worked with and call those models for references. Ask them for a business card. In other words, do everything possible to make sure they are legitimate. Find out if you can take someone with you on the shoot. If they say "no," that is a good indication you don't want to work with them. *Note:* When Shannon started out, she took someone with her to most of her bookings or testings. Now she feels confident with her screening process. Even if she doesn't take someone along, she often asks if she can to see how the photographer will react. She always takes someone with her if she doesn't feel 100 percent certain about a booking.

Shannon networks with other cyber models, and her Web page includes links to their sites. Although agencies sometimes contact her wanting to represent her, she declines because she enjoys working on her own.

At the time Shannon was interviewed for this book, her Web site was getting between 35,000 and 45,000 hits per day, and she was receiving around three hundred e-mails per day. Part of Shannon's success is attributed to the fact that she has put together a great Web site. She taught herself the art of Web design, using a "What You See Is What You Get" (WYSIWYG) application in the beginning. Now she is fluent in HTML. She updates her site about once per month, three times a month in the summer.

If you are interested in promoting yourself as a model through your own Web site, there are plenty of resources to help you get started. Most Internet service providers offer free Web sites and have tutorials for step-by-step Web-site creation. Once you get up and running, though, you will need your own domain name for a more professional image.

Finding Photographers on the Web

There are plenty of professional photographers who have Web sites, and the Internet has become a great way for models and photographers to connect. In chapter 20 you will find Web-site information that will help you find photographers. Be sure you ask for and check references–don't be afraid to ask photographers for the names and phone numbers of at least two models with whom they have worked. Photographers should not object if you ask to bring along a chaperone; however, as mentioned before, it is your responsibility to make sure the chaperone is one that will not get in the way or make anyone on the set uncomfortable.

CHAPTER FOURTEEN

The Business Basics

"Yesterday is a cancelled check; tomorrow is a promissory note;
today is the only cash you have—so spend it wisely."

KAY LYONS

*A*lthough keeping up with receipts, preparing taxes, and managing money can be a dull part of a model's life, it can determine whether you succeed or fail. Models often have to depend on their savings to get through the lean times, when they have few or no bookings. Models are also considered independent contractors, so they are therefore responsible for keeping up with their income and expenses and reporting and paying their taxes. Agencies do not withhold or help models prepare taxes or pay for benefits such as health insurance. These responsibilities are placed solely on the model.

As soon as you start to earn money, find an accountant to help you with tax preparation, record keeping, and investments. Ask your agency if it can recommend any Certified Public Accountants (CPAs) and get recommendations from other models or people you know and trust. Interview several CPAs before you decide on an accountant. Find out what each accountant's experience is in preparing tax returns for individuals who are models, actors, or entertainment professionals. Ask if the accountant will make herself available if you are be audited in the future. Compare the accountant's fees and find out if she can recommend a system to help you maintain your income and expense records, and if she will counsel you on appropriate deductible expenses.

Taxes

Even after you hire an accountant, you are ultimately responsible for the proper filing of your state and federal tax returns. Each year, your agency will send you a Form 1099, which reports your earnings. Since you are considered an independent contractor, agencies do not take out taxes from your pay. Basically, you don't work for the agency–you work for yourself. Your CPA can save you time and money, but the burden of maintaining records and filing taxes on time rests on your shoulders. Taking care of such business matters is not that difficult, but you do need to be organized and informed. Well-maintained, updated records will help make these tasks a lot easier.

As a model, you are technically in business for yourself, so you will need to learn how to track your tax-deductible expenses. In order to do so effectively, you need to stay on top of new tax laws that govern allowable expenses. Your accountant will be able to give you advice on deductible expenses and help you devise a system that will best suit your needs. It could be something as simple as keeping an envelope for receipts of each type of expense (like supplies, travel, prints, composites, etc.) to putting this information on a personal computer. If you have a computer, there are some simple bookkeeping programs, like Quicken, that can simplify your record keeping. Such programs track your deductible expenses and help you keep your accounts balanced.

Pertinent information should be indicated on your receipts, and you should keep these receipts organized, particularly receipts for expenses more than $25. For example, if you pay for the reprinting of composite cards, your receipt should indicate the date the expense occurred, the amount of the expense, the name of the company or vendor, an explanation of what was purchased (three hundred composite cards), and the method of payment (cash, credit card, check).

Expenses that involve meals or entertainment should include the name(s) of the individual(s) you treated as well as the purpose of the expense. An example would be taking out a makeup artist for dinner after a shoot. If you discuss business, this would be a deductible expense. Examples of other allowable deductions include:

- Photographers' fees.
- Prints, composites from photography.
- Cost of duplicate prints for portfolio.
- Composite-card printing.
- Portfolio case.
- Demo tape production and duplication.
- Cost involved for representation in agency's promotional materials.
- Stationery or any office supplies needed to organize or maintain your business.
- Appointment book.
- Telephone costs (phone line, answering machine, pager, beeper, cell phone, answering service, computer line).
- Nonreimbursed commuting or transportation cost involved with your work. (This does not include going to your agency, but only to appointments, go-sees, and modeling jobs.) This includes airfare, cab fare (plus tips), subway or bus fare, car rentals, and mileage.
- Entertainment, such as attending an event that will enhance your career or that will help you gain knowledge in your field. (For example, the admission to a fashion show.)
- Items of clothing or accessories specifically required for your work. Naturally, this does not include items you purchase that are later reimbursed by the client.
- The services of hair and makeup professionals.
- Cosmetics and toiletries purchased for your modeling case.
- The preparation and printing of your résumé.
- Commissions paid to your agency.
- Union dues and membership fees (for example, the Screen Actors

Guild [SAG], the American Federation of Television and Radio Artists [AFTRA] national labor union, and the Model's Guild).
- Legal, bookkeeping, and tax-preparation fees.
- Magazines and books that relate to your field, if they are necessary
in continuing your knowledge of the business.

The Model's Guild

Don't count on your agency for health insurance; most agencies treat
their models as independent contractors who are responsible for their
own health care. This is another reason why you might consider the
Model's Guild. The organization has minimal eligibility requirements. To
join, you only need to show proof of having been paid for at least two
professional jobs within the past year. National Health Care plans are
offered at a reasonable rate, and membership is also open to other fashion industry professionals such as agents, photographers, make-up artists, and hair stylists.

The Guild, which was established in 1995 to help protect models and
offer them benefits, also offers general modeling advice. If you live and
work in New York, you can attend Guild workshops designed to help
models at all levels of the profession. Contact the Model's Guild at 265
West 14th Street, New York, NY 10011, (800) 864-4696 or (212) 675-4133.

Making Ends Meet

If you don't have a significant amount of resources to sustain your living
expenses when you first begin your modeling career, you will probably
need to supplement your income. Models work part-time jobs, waitress,
or sign up with temporary employment agencies to help make ends meet.

Temporary employment agencies are ideal for earning extra money
without committing to a full-time schedule, especially if you have cleri-
cal skills. Even if you don't have office or computer skills, you can work
through a temporary agency as a receptionist or file clerk. In major metropolitan areas, there are many temporary agencies to choose from, and
once you register, you choose what days you want to work. One more

added benefit is that you will have an opportunity to learn more about computers and software programs and see a variety of different businesses. Whether you end up working as a full-time model or not, the skills you learn could be of tremendous benefit to many areas of your life.

If you decide to work part-time, select jobs that offer flexibility or afternoon/early evening schedules that will free up your days for go-sees, castings, testings, and other appointments. Do not select a part-time job that will keep you out too late. Having dark circles under your eyes and arriving at go-sees with a yawn could adversely effect your career.

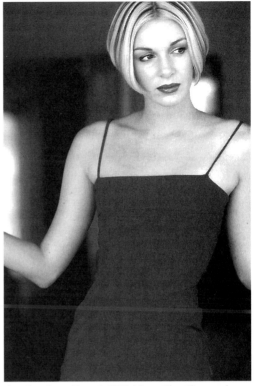

Photo by Johnny Olsen. © 1999 Johnny Olsen Photography.

Preparing and Living within a Budget

If you are new to New York, you may be amazed at how fast you go through money. From taxicabs to grabbing a sandwich at the local deli, expenses can escalate. Get a handle on how much you are spending by looking at a month's worth of expenses. List how much you paid for rent, transportation, utilities, groceries, restaurants, hair care, wardrobe, accessories, and modeling expenses (i.e., prints, cards, or testings). After reviewing your spending habits, you may be surprised to learn how much you spend on things like eating out or taxis. How much could you save in one month if you took the subway? Would that be enough to help pay for a testing? If your finances are tight, find ways to cut back and work toward saving money.

Savings

When you start working as a model on a regular basis, develop the habit of putting a set amount aside as savings. When you work in a profession that does not pay on a regular basis, your survival could depend on your ability to save money. It takes a lot of discipline, but it is wise to start saving from the very beginning. Even if you start making a lot of money, if you've developed a good habit of saving, you'll be able to accumulate a substantially larger amount.

Investing in Your Career

As a model, there are certain costs you will incur on a regular basis. You will need to build and maintain your portfolio, keep your looks updated, invest in wardrobe, and maintain a supply of composite cards. These expenses are ongoing, and in the beginning, you might find that they absorb most of your income. Consider these expenses a necessary part of building a career. Since most of these expenses are tax–deductible, they will help offset your income.

Model Contracts

Most agencies will request that you sign a contract, and since most agencies expect you to commit to a period of time in exchange for their investment in helping to get your career off the ground, it stands to reason that these agreements are exclusive. The time period can range from one year to five years. Since the early 1990s, many new agencies have opened, and there has been fierce competition among agents. Models are lured from one agency to the next. Contracts are broken, fees and commission agreements are renegotiated, and new contracts are signed.

You don't have to sign a contract, and you certainly have the option to change the terms if you feel your needs will not be met under the terms specified. Some contracts are very simple and serve to protect both you and the agency. Some basic information included in a contract is as follows:

- The agency agrees to represent you and help you obtain work. (Basically, you are hiring the agency to work for you.)
- If the contract is an exclusive agreement, you agree to utilize only the agency (or its representatives) to obtain modeling assignments. In a nonexclusive agreement, you may procure assignments through other sources.
- The agency commission or fee (usually 20 percent) and the duration of the contract is stipulated.

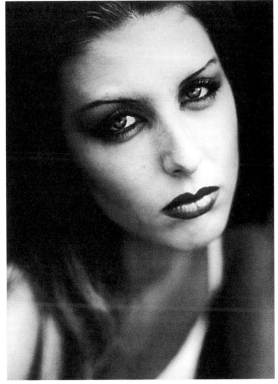

Photo by Jason Perkins. © Jason Perkins.
Model: Amy, Grant Models, Calgary.

You should feel very comfortable with your agency and not have any doubts about it representing you. If you are not totally comfortable, you could request that a ninety–day trial period be written into the contract. Talk over the terms and conditions with your parents, other models, and an attorney, and make the most well–informed decision you can.

CHAPTER FIFTEEN

Careers in Fashion and Related Industries

"Success in highest and noblest form calls for peace of mind and enjoyment and happiness, which comes only to the man who has found the work he likes best."

NAPOLEON HILL

For several reasons, this could be one of the most important chapters in this book. It is valuable to be knowledgeable about the various professions in the modeling industry. Obviously you're interested in this industry, or you would have never picked up this book.

By now, you have an idea of how difficult and competitive modeling can be. Remember, modeling isn't right for everyone, and you should always be aware of your options. It is to your benefit to have some alternative paths in mind in case you find (for whatever reason) modeling is not for you. Even if you become a model, it helps to understand how everything comes together behind the scenes in the creation of fashion shows, advertising campaigns, or magazines. Learning something about the people who labor "backstage" will help you build a strong foundation in the profession and appreciate those individuals for the work that they do.

There are so many exciting opportunities available for those who want to pursue a career in the fashion industry. Even if you become a successful model, you need to plan for the possibility of your career losing momentum as you get older. It is important to establish long-term goals. It's been said that modeling lasts about fifteen minutes, which might be what it feels like to a lot of models who are fading out of the business. Whether you plan to model for a year, five years, or forty years, it can't hurt to know about the careers of your coworkers in the industry.

Acting

Acting is one of the most competitive fields one can try to break into, but a lot of models have set their sights on an acting career. If that is what you think you want, you must have a burning desire to pursue acting as a career and go after it with all you've got. Do your homework. Get a degree in theater. Move to a major metropolitan area (if you don't already live in one). And develop a very thick skin, at least in dealing with rejection.

Agent/Booker

Most model agents, or bookers, start out as employees in modeling agencies and work their way up. A booker is responsible for promoting models, booking work, negotiating fees, and building a model's career. Bookers must maintain good relationships with clients and be able to hammer out all the details between the model and client. The booker interfaces with photographers, editors, and clients and essentially acts as a salesperson for the model. Since bookers are usually responsible for the scheduling and management of several models, this profession comes with a significant amount of stress, so bookers must have an outgoing personality, be energetic, and be very well organized. Another requirement is a passion for the fashion business and an eye for recognizing a model's potential.

You can also find bookers who work for magazines, and they are responsible for booking models, makeup artists, and other professionals for a layout. In addition, agencies who represent other artists (i.e., photographers, makeup artists, hairstylists) also hire bookers.

This profession does not require formal training. If you decide to become an agent after being a model, you already have a working knowledge of the business and can empathize with models. Great agents are very much in demand and can earn decent six-figure salaries. In fact, top agents are often wined and dined by competing firms in hopes of persuading them to switch agencies.

Photographer

To establish a career as a photographer, one must have a combination of technical expertise and artistic ability. Most photographers have a specific style, just like painters or designers. Once a photographer has achieved success and/or notoriety, his work is easily recognized because of his unique style. Some photographers attend colleges that offer art programs or obtain basic technical skills through classes or workshops, while others begin as photographer's assistants and work their way up.

While some photographers set up their own studios and work independently, it is also possible to establish a career as an in-house photographer working for catalog companies, corporations, publications, or studios.

Photography equipment is very expensive, so setting up a studio requires capital. Other expenses involved in this profession include a portfolio and composite cards. Although this field is highly skilled and artistic, several models have successfully made the transition to photography.

Fashion Designer

For a career as a fashion designer, you should have a strong artistic background. Most designers are able to sketch out their designs and put together garments, which involves creating a pattern, sewing, and draping. One way to get started in this field is to work as an apprentice (or designer's assistant). Some designers create designs for apparel companies and others create their own. Successful independent designers employ a number of people and often manufacture their garments.

Fashion Writers and Editors for Magazines and Trades

If you enjoy reading and looking through fashion magazines and you're good at writing, you might want to consider a career with a fashion publication. Take a look at any major magazine's masthead (the list of the people who put out the magazine), and you'll discover a lot of professionals behind those glossy, colorful pages. There are positions such as fashion writers, art directors, beauty editors, design directors, copy editors, assistants, beauty directors, research associates, and production directors—just to name a few. If you are interested in working in any of these positions, it is suggested that you obtain a college degree in journalism, English, or business administration. Another way to break in is to start as a secretary or clerk and work your way up. Keep in mind that magazine or advertising jobs are generally not the best-paying jobs, at least in the beginning. For instance, if you start out as a secretary for a magazine, you might not earn as much money as a secretary who works for an investment bank.

Fashion Stylist

This artistic individual must be a whiz at putting together clothes, accessories, and props and be very organized and detail-oriented. She can work independently or be represented by an agent. Requirements vary from being self-taught and talented in style to a background in fashion design or art.

Makeup Artist

If you love makeup, enjoy working with people, and can fully appreciate the artistry that goes into creating a new face with the use of makeup technique, you might want to consider this profession. Depending on where you live, in order to work as a professional makeup artist you might need to obtain a state-approved license after attending cosmetology school. A license may not be required in every state, so be sure to investigate the legal requirements in the city where you plan to work.

The cost of schools and the required amount of time varies from state to state. You might want to find a school where you can major in makeup artistry rather than pick it up as part of regular cosmetology curriculum. Some professionals suggest that you work at one of the makeup shops or cosmetic counters where you can network with other people in the industry.

A makeup artist puts together a portfolio that demonstrates his/her talent and skill as well as a composite card, which is used to attract and build the artist's business. Your clients will be photographers, agencies, and other companies that use makeup artists. There are agents who represent makeup artists, but some artists choose to work independently. (For information regarding training and books on this subject, see chapter 20.)

~

From Modeling to Making Up

Sherrie Long made the transformation from model to professional makeup artist. In a brief interview, she shared a few thoughts on how she switched careers:

Press: Why did you switch careers from model to makeup artist?
Sherrie: We all travel a long journey to our chosen career. But to sum it all up, I got tired of working with really bad makeup artists. By *bad,* I mean unsanitary (using the same mascara on every one of the models, or using the same makeup sponge on everyone's skin) and untrained (hired because they said they knew what they were doing or hired because they were a friend of the designers).

I think another reason models become

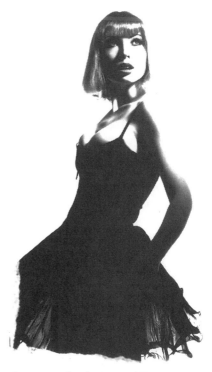

Sherrie Long. Photo by Kingmond Young.

makeup artists is because as a model, you work with agencies. You never really feel fully in charge of your own career. As a makeup artist, you are in charge. You book your own clients and develop closeness professionally with the clients, which you were not allowed to do as a model.

Press: How did you train to become a makeup artist?
Sherrie: As a model, I would be asked to apply the other models' makeup when it was apparent the makeup artist hired for that day didn't know what he was doing. As a result, I went to school in Los Angeles to study makeup professionally. I pride myself for being exceptionally clean, professional, and well trained.

Press: What do you like best about your career?
Sherrie: Creativity, and knowing that I am in charge of my own career. As a makeup artist, there is no game playing. You get in, do your job, and leave. You don't have to charm anyone.

~

Hairstylist

Depending on what city you plan to work in, if you want to be a hairstylist you may be required to be licensed though a state-accredited cosmetology school. To work as a hairstylist for models doing fashion-magazine or runway work, you need to be extremely versatile and artistic. Just like models, top hairstylists of this type work through an agency. These artists have their own promotional materials, such as a portfolio filled with tear sheets as well as composite cards, that exhibit their work.

Stylist

Do you have a talent for putting together colors, clothing, jewelry, hats, shoes, scarves, and belts? Do you like to create a look that is unique and stylish? If so, this might be a career to consider. The stylist usually selects the clothing and entire ensemble, including props and accessories. Stylists can either work freelance, through an agency, or for a magazine.

Broadcasting

If you are interested in a broadcasting career, such as a news anchorperson or weather personality, you'll need to have a great voice and be very comfortable working in front of a camera. Most individuals who work in these fields have earned a college degree and have started out by working as an intern for a television station.

Artist's Representative/Agent

Artist's representatives work in the same way model agents work in that they obtain assignments or contracts for their artists and charge a percentage of fees billed to the clients. As mentioned before, makeup artists, photographers, and hairstylists can choose to utilize a representative in the same way a model does.

Advertising

Probably one of the best ways to begin a career in advertising is as a college intern. There are various positions available in the advertising field; some possible choices are account executive, researcher, art director, casting director, copywriter, or in production. You could even work with computers or digital imagery. Karl Rudisill is president and CEO of DICE, a digital composite company in New York. Karl started out with an engineering background but found professional success as a model. He came to Manhattan–after spending time modeling in Europe for the Ford Agency–with "an idea and a suitcase" and went on to become a photographer. Finally, he combined all of his talents into his current venture: a high-quality, very creative digital-imagery company.

Public Relations

A career in public relations can be exciting for those who love to interact with people and are great at promotion. A variety of skills are needed to work in "PR," including communicating well, both orally and in writing;

organizing pertinent promotional materials; engaging the media and draw-ing its attention to the client; and hosting promotional events such as parties or receptions. Public-relations professionals can choose to work for a company or work independently.

Set Designer

This professional designs sets for photo shoots, live promotions, fashion shows, and media events, selecting colors, themes, locations, necessary props, and so on. This individual must be very detail-oriented, energetic, and talented in terms of seeing a project through from concept to reality, working closely with photographers, clients, directors, and most every-one else involved in production.

No matter what career you choose following your modeling days (if any), it will only be as much fun as you make it. Who knows? Even if you become a modeling superstar, you may still find there are greater, more exciting horizons ahead.

CHAPTER SIXTEEN

Advice for Concerned Parents

*"Expect trouble as an inevitable part of life and repeat to yourself
the most comforting words of all: 'This, too, shall pass.'"*

ANN LANDERS

$\mathcal{I}$t wasn't until several years after I had moved to New York that my father confessed how much he worried about my working and living in Manhattan. Now, as a mother of a young girl, I can imagine how I'd feel if my daughter wanted to move to New York at age sixteen (or younger) to pursue modeling—and I did so when I was in my early twenties. It is important that you investigate and understand the modeling industry in order to guide your child in the right direction. I honestly don't expect to diminish your worries and fears but hope to give you knowledge and suggestions as to how you can guide your young model to a lucrative, successful, but most importantly, safe career.

Teens in the Adult Market

You, as legal guardian, are the one who will ultimately determine if a modeling career is something you want your child to pursue. By "child,"

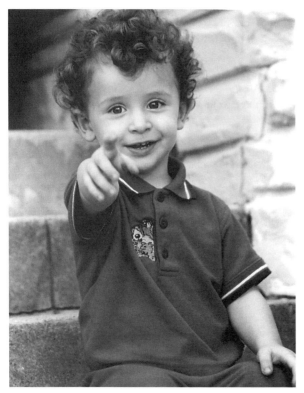

Photo by Erin Ashley.

I am referring to a minor (between the ages of thirteen and seventeen) and not a young child (ages six months to twelve years). Although young children are discussed at the end of this chapter, most of the information herein pertains to underage models who work in the adult market.

You might be surprised to learn that it is typical for agencies to represent thirteen-year-olds who model in the adult/women's market. These girls may look mature for their age after they are "made up," primarily because of their height. Models in this category tend to be around 5'8" tall, and most of the younger ones have not finished growing. If you examine some of the print work that these models produce, you can't help but notice that they are indeed very young teens made to look like adults. Often you will see prints of them in evening wear, something low cut or sheer, and you can tell that they are so young, they've not yet developed breasts.

A Look at Agencies

If you have a very young child who wants to model, and an agency is knocking on your door to represent her, ask to see the agency's book. This book contains all of the print work/composites of the models the agency represents. Determine whether or not you can picture your "child" in this environment, posing for pictures like the ones you see in the book. If you don't have access to an agency book, look for it on the Internet. Most major agencies have Web sites that show prints of their models.

Starting Out

I personally believe that models (in the adult market) should not be younger than age eighteen, and I am not alone in my opinion. I met with numerous top professionals in the industry who told me the same thing over and over: "We don't like the fact that we start models out as young as age thirteen, but if we don't take them, someone else will."

Michele Persinger, formerly with Elite LA, started modeling at thirteen years old. She ended up working in the Asian market in Osaka and Kobe. The fact that she was home schooled certainly helped. "There were a lot of girls my age who dropped out of school to model. I was fortunate to have the support of my family behind me, who encouraged me to continue with my home schooling." Although Michele is appreciative of her opportunity to model, she believes that thirteen is too young to model away from home. "There are far too many temptations–and since most drop out of school, when their modeling career is over, they don't know what to do."

One option for starting at such a young age is to try the business out in the summer or on spring/fall breaks from school. A lot of models get started this way. They don't miss school, and they get an introduction to the exciting world of modeling. This is possible for those who live near the major markets and can easily access the agency (and the work) during breaks and summer vacation. Wendy Rose of Ford works with clients who live "within a one-hour commute of New York. That way, if we call them for a go-see, they can be there quickly. And if they decide not to take the job because of a school commitment, that's okay, too. There are plenty of models who live within this radius to contact for the go-see or booking, so it isn't a problem. The child can enjoy modeling as well as a normal life."

One possible downfall is when the model goes back to school; she may find that she can't relate as well to others. If Sally has earned $1,500 per day all summer long, it may be hard for her friend Mary to relate, since Mary has been waiting tables all summer, lucky to earn $100 per day.

Trusting Your Teenage Model

Ultimately, we have to trust our youngsters to remain levelheaded and not make unwise or unsafe choices. My father always told me, "Use your own good judgment in everything you do." I actually thought of those words when faced with some choices that could have spelled disaster. Of course, I made my own choices and my own mistakes, but I always felt as if I had a guiding light. My parents instilled in me a solid base of values. Although I encountered plenty of opportunities to mess up my life, I ultimately ended up making the right choices. Various individuals in the business have cited this very issue as one of the most important things to consider when it comes to a minor pursuing a modeling career–from what type of family or home base does she come? Monique Pillard, president of Elite, has probably seen more modeling successes and failures than anyone in the business, and she wholeheartedly agrees. "This profession is much easier if the girl has a very happy and good family life," she advises. "Most successful models who enjoy a healthy career come from a very stable family."

Managing Your Young Model's Career

You should be involved and included in all meetings between your child and the agency representative, understanding as much as possible about the business before giving the green light for your child to pursue modeling. It is very important that you carefully read and understand chapter 10, which covers scams and some of the pitfalls that can happen when you don't know how this business works. This information will help you detect unprofessional individuals, businesses, and scam artists. When you are faced with a questionable situation, you (the parent or guardian) can usually make an objective judgment. After all, the young model's dream is hanging in the balance, and her judgment could well be clouded.

You should feel very comfortable with the agency that represents your son or daughter. The agency should be available to answer all of the questions you might have and should be able to give you firsthand information about assignments, travel arrangements, housing arrangements, financial matters, and so on. There should never be a problem with you accompanying your child to a work location, testing, or agency appointment. As the parent of a minor, the agency should make you feel good about being involved and not hesitate to include you in decision making.

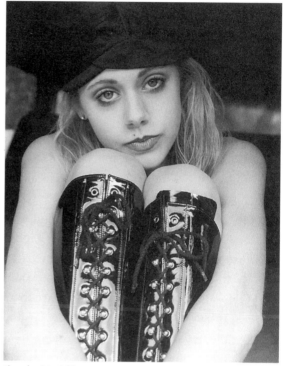

Photo by Erin Ashley.

Parents should not rush into signing a contract with an agency and should first meet with all interested agencies. There is no reason to race to sign a contract with the first agency that offers; if the agency is interested now, it will be a month from now. You can also exercise the option to not sign a contract. Depending on your financial situation, the agency may only allow advances to get started (for testings, portfolio, travel, relocation) if you obligate to a specified amount of time by signing a contract. Even if money is advanced, you can sign an agreement to pay back advances out of the model's earnings.

If you do decide to sign a contract with an agency, make sure you have a clear understanding as to the financial terms. You should also know what expenses will be billed on the model's behalf. (Refer to chapter 7 for more information involving reasonable costs incurred by the model.)

Parents should not only meet with the agency representative, but with the booker who will be working for the model. The booker is the main contact person your child will have in the modeling world, so make sure you have good rapport with him or her.

Education

When it comes to education, I hope most parents will agree that it shouldn't be sacrificed for a modeling career. Far too many models find themselves at the ripe old age of twenty-three with no money, no skills or knowledge in any field but modeling, and no education. They feel very insecure in the real world. No matter what type of student your child is, basic education should not be put on the back burner. Parents should be very active in monitoring home or professional schooling to make sure that education doesn't take second place to modeling.

If at all possible, try to inspire your child to expand her education while traveling, which tends to help tremendously when models maintain other interests. If she has an interest in art, she might take a class in art history while in Paris. Expanding her interests outside the world of modeling will help to keep her grounded.

Travel

Would you have a problem sending your sixteen-year-old to New York to live and work alone? I am amazed to hear how often young models are not chaperoned. Gideon Lewin, a well-known fashion photographer, shared with me how he had a fourteen-year-old model show up at his studio alone. He called the agency to request that they immediately send over a chaperone. "Parents should be concerned about bringing very young teens into this business," Gideon offers. Most top professionals in the business agree, but unfortunately, there are no set standards regulating this industry. All too often, very young girls are thrown in the middle of this adult world and expected to swim on their own, whether they're in Europe or New York.

The bottom line is, don't assume your child will be supervised or chaperoned, even if you've been told that she will. Unless the model is an overnight sensation and of superstar caliber, she won't be chaperoned unless you make those arrangements. A parent or guardian should plan to travel with the model. You can't rely on the agencies to provide chaperones, and in all fairness, they don't have the staff to function in this capacity. From time to time, you'll find an agent who will chaperone a model, but for the most part, this does not occur.

Coping with Change

Depending on who the models are and their backgrounds and support systems, many of them get spoiled and seemingly change overnight. All of a sudden, they find they are making a lot of money and are working as adults, yet their agent(s) and parents still tell them what to do. They begin to resent these authority figures. Here they are, thrown into an adult environment where the stakes are high, and everyone is continuously making a fuss over them. They are pulled at, pushed, and driven to "ride the waves as long as the surf is up." It is easy to see how they can lose perspective as to what's really important. It is a lot to expect that someone so young will be able to handle this type of life and come out unscathed, and it is easy to understand how someone without a strong network of support can be ruined in one way or another.

It is not impossible for a thirteen-year-old to work in this business without going down the wrong path, but based on numerous interviews with top professionals, open and honest communication as to what this business can *really* be like is a must for parents with children who model.

Money Management

Just as with adult models, sometimes it takes six or seven months to start making money. When models begin earning a lot of money, they tend to want a place of their own and no longer want to stay in the models' apartments. Apartments in New York are certainly not cheap, so these models may find they are paying for space they are not fully utilizing. Beginning models often travel so much they end up spending half of their time away from home. Spending can get out of control fast. Instead of living modestly and saving money, a model may spend her income as fast as it is earned. Then, before she knows it, she ages and finds that she is no longer in such hot demand, basically having nothing to show for years of effort–no skills, no education, and no savings.

Parents should, if at all possible, monitor the model's spending and teach her the value of money. They should encourage her to save and invest, occasionally bringing her back down to earth with the reminder that she probably won't earn money like that forever. They should encourage her to be conservative and suggest that she share an apartment with two or three other models. Depending on the city, they might advise her to investigate a women's-only residence or boardinghouse. Another option is to suggest that the model consider roommates who are outside of the modeling world, which might provide a more stable environment.

Parents should help their model figure out how much of her earnings to save and what she can spend. The savings account will help when the model hits dry periods and business slows down, which can easily happen in the fashion industry. Once the model starts to make money, it is wise to find a trustworthy financial advisor who is not directly connected with her agency. Parents may opt to give the model a living allowance and put the remainder into an investment account where the money can't be readily accessed.

Parents should also stay on top of the model's career and help prepare her for the day she is no longer making money. If you guide her to be smart with her money, this transition will certainly be a lot easier.

Homesickness

One of the problems experienced by young models, particularly those away from home for the first time, is that they end up spending a lot of time alone. All of a sudden, they find that they are in a foreign land or a new city with no friends. It is lonely, scary, and incredibly intimidating. They may develop short–term relationships, but unfortunately, there's not enough time spent in one place to develop long–lasting ones. Sadly enough, when the model communicates with her friends and family from home, she finds that they're continuing with their lives and relation-ships, and she starts to feel left out. This type of thing can put a lot of pressure on a girl. Frankly, it can break her, sometimes leading to depres-sion, drinking, or drugs.

Final Thoughts on Teens and Modeling

While interviewing top professionals for this book, I found two interest-ing facts that cannot be overlooked. First, I asked: "If you had a daughter, would you encourage her to model?" An overwhelming majority indi-cated that they would. The second question I asked was: "Do you know of some truly happy models who really have it together?" Most people hesitated for a long period of time, struggling to find one or two names. Even a few successful models indicated that they did not know of many "truly happy" individuals who are models. The models perceived as "happy" have the same traits: They come from good homes with a strong family background (with which they maintain a solid connection), and they do not take their careers too seriously. (In other words, they have other interests.)

Don't expect to enter your child into this profession as a means to boost her confidence. Typically, the opposite occurs because of the high level of rejection a model must withstand. It's a highly competitive busi-ness, and very, very few make it to the top. It is bad enough to suffer occasional rejection as a teenager, but to experience it on a daily basis is very tough on the ego. This business is known for being brutal. It doesn't matter that the kid is only fourteen years old–there are rude people in this business who don't discriminate according to age. These types of individuals and the poisonous messages they dish out can be disastrous to fragile young minds.

From Babies to Young Teens

Unlike teen models, child models are not subject to the potential pitfalls and dangers discussed above. Child models (babies, toddlers, young chil-dren, and young teens) who are represented by a reputable agent are usually able to pursue modeling with minimal problems. Their parents or a guardian are with them at all times, and they continue their education. Modeling is treated as an extracurricular activity; the kids have a lot of fun and generally find the overall experience rewarding. If your young child wants to model and you live in a city where this option is feasible, there is generally no need for concern–providing you have engaged a well-known, reputable agent. (See chapter 3 for more information about child models and chapter 10 for information on scams and unethical practices.)

Young teens can also model in a branch of the children's division that also covers the teen market. According to Wendy Rose from the Ford agency in New York, Ford has a small teen division that represents teens who are marketed *as teens*. These girls are usually shorter and have a younger look than girls of the same age who are placed in the regular adult division.

Your child will not need photographs or a portfolio in order to find an agent. Take a snapshot or two to an agency's open call or send them to the agency along with the child's age, height, weight, eye color, and hair color. Children three years of age and older have professional headshots taken after they sign with an agency. The agency will recommend several photographers, but the decision will ultimately be up to the parents. The cost for a photo session can range from $100 to $500. Once a year, your child's photo will be placed in the agency's headshot book at a cost of $200 to $250. These expenses are to be expected in this business, even for children. Children's looks change frequently, so the composite card must be updated more frequently than for a conventional adult model.

Children who model fashion for a major New York agency must live within reasonable proximity to the city, generally within a one–hour commute, in order to take advantage of go–sees and last–minute bookings. This would apply in any major city.

As mentioned before, a child's education should never be sacrificed in any way for a modeling career. If an agency represents children, you'll find they represent a lot of kids. Because of school schedules and a child's inability to work constantly, agencies need many children to fulfill their clients' needs. Children can pursue modeling in the summer or during spring or fall break, or in conjunction with home schooling or tutoring if they are working steadily.

When a child model loses a tooth, he will probably need to invest in a "flipper" tooth, which is a false tooth that is "flipped" in for a shoot. The flipper tooth must be adjusted as the child's tooth grows.

A child's income from modeling should never be relied upon for family support. Unfortunately, some parents push their kids into a modeling career because of the child's earning potential. This puts an incredible amount of pressure on the child, which is unfair. When money is paid to the child, it is issued in the child's name, and earnings should be deposited into a guardian account until the child reaches age eighteen. However, there are no strict guidelines that govern this process. A child model, like other models, is considered an independent contractor, and she will need her own social security number and be expected to pay estimated taxes.

Parents should feel positive about their relationship with their child's agent, be willing to rely on the agency's judgment, and feel confident their child is getting the best representation. Parents might hear about a casting call and wonder why their blonde-haired, blue-eyed Bonnie didn't get to go on the go-see, only to learn that the agent didn't send Bonnie because the call was for a brunette. A good representative will not waste a child's time on a go-see that the child doesn't have a chance of booking.

When it comes to child modeling, the most important thing to consider is whether your child really wants to do this type of work. Modeling is a great way for kids to have fun while earning money, but if the child isn't enjoying the work, don't push him or her into the business.

CHAPTER SEVENTEEN

Training

*"You only grow by coming to the end of something
and by beginning something else."*

JOHN IRVING

$\mathcal{M}$ost agencies and industry professionals do not advocate modeling schools. The standard belief in this industry is that you don't need to have previous training or to attend modeling school in order to work as a model. Nevertheless, there are schools that are reputable and have helped models launch successful careers. It is true–if you have what it takes, you can become a successful model without going through any formal training. But since some modeling schools offer exposure and introductions to agencies and plan trips to New York or other major markets, for some individuals it makes the investment worthwhile. Modeling schools also plan group trips to modeling conventions and scout for major agencies. If you want to pursue modeling as a career but don't feel as if you are ready to pack your bags and head for New York, a good, reputable modeling school might be a good stepping–stone.

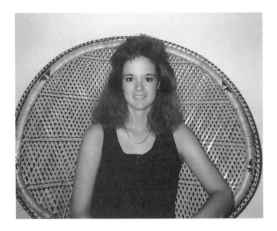

Role-Model School

There are not many modeling schools that are viewed favorably by agencies, but one school stands out. Nancy Bounds Studios, Inc., located in Omaha, Nebraska, is regularly mentioned in a very favorable way among industry professionals in New York. Because of the good reputation of this school, I've highlighted it as our "role-model" school, which is the type of school you should try to find where you live.

Nancy Bounds Studios is incorporated and is regulated and authorized to operate by the Commissioner of Education of the state of Nebraska. Courses begin every month and are two hours long, held once a week for thirty weeks. The facility provides training areas and equipment for runway, photo/television viewing and taping, dressing rooms, a makeup area, and lecture rooms. Equipment includes still and video cameras, VCR and monitor, professional lighting, spotlights, stereo tape recorders, CD player, and a computer to help track students and models worldwide.

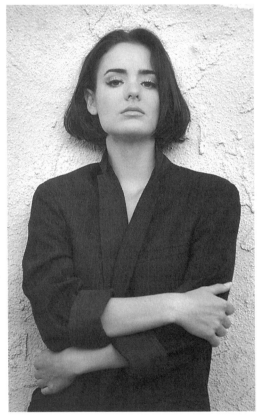

All photos, this and facing page, courtesy Nancy Bounds Studio.

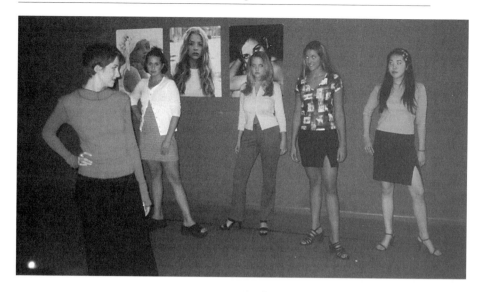

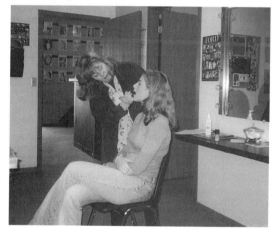

The highly refined course was developed over the past thirty years and is always evolving. The curriculum is original, copyrighted, and widely respected within the industry, the objective of which is to make students look their best and achieve self- and social confidence. Naturally, grooming is a part of the course. It includes figure control, hair care, hairstyling, skin care, makeup, fashion knowledge, and developing an individual sense of style. Professional modeling techniques are interwoven throughout the course.

Two written tests are administered, one at the fifteenth and another at the thirtieth week. Two visual tests and as many as ten "pop quizzes" are possible. Students are also graded on their notebooks, which contain:

- Notes from class
- Extracurricular homework and research on subjects relevant to class material

- Pictures taken from fashion publications that reflect "do's and don'ts" of wardrobe, visual poise, hair, and so on.
- Evaluations
- Model manners for job interviews and go–sees
- Valuable handouts, which are updated regularly to keep students current on fashion and industry trends
- Notes and breakdowns of all model movements; i.e., runway, photo, and TV commercials

Progress reports to students are made verbally, and parent/teacher conferences are encouraged. If a student does not graduate for reasons of unsatisfactory progress, he or she will be invited to restudy all or part of the course free of charge. Throughout the year, national and international scouts and agents visit Nancy Bounds Studios, who meet with graduates with professional model potential.

Enrollment procedures involve a meeting with the Admissions Department. Parents are requested to attend this meeting if the student is younger than nineteen. The prospective student should be prepared to speak about her goals and how she thinks the school might help her reach these goals. There are no high–pressure sales tactics at Nancy Bounds Studios and no obligation involved with the interview process.

Great emphasis is placed on placement at Nancy Bounds Studios for local, national, and international modeling opportunities. Graduates from this school are working professionally in places like New York, Paris, Milan, Hamburg, Munich, Madrid, Tokyo, Osaka, San Francisco, and Miami Beach. Many others are employed in fashion retail, merchandising, advertising, fashion coordination, makeup, hairstyling, and other related fields.

Potential models are encouraged to do testings and build a portfolio. Once the model's book is of professional quality, she is encouraged to make go–sees to important local clients. Graduates are exposed to top agencies, and when the time comes, they are assisted with contracts, lodging, passports, visas, tickets, taxes, and customs.

Nancy Bounds Studios is located at 11915 Pierce Plaza, Omaha, NE 68144; (402) 697-9292.

Finding a Modeling School

A reputable modeling school should teach:

- Poise
- Confidence
- Professionalism
- Grooming
- Rejection acceptance
- Posing
- Runway techniques
- Informal modeling
- Professional makeup technique
- Television–commercial work

Before investing in a modeling school, find out how much it will cost. Think about the value of the curriculum offered and the exposure to agents versus what you can obtain on your own. Ask the school director about the teachers and their level of experience. Find out if any of their students have achieved success as models. Does the school offer work–shops conducted by industry professionals, such as a runway trainer or professional makeup artist? Does it offer agency contact opportunities?

If you want to attend a modeling school, it is advisable to visit as many schools as you can and compare them against these guidelines. Follow the same guidelines in investigating a school as you would with an agency. If the school is one that you have not heard much about, call the Better Business Bureau and ask if they have had any complaints. Ask the schools you visit if you can sit in on a class. Most schools should not have a problem with this request, and auditing a class will help you to evaluate the school's potential to fit your needs.

CHAPTER EIGHTEEN

Conventions and Contests

"Satisfaction lies in the effort, not in the attainment.
Full effort is full victory."

MAHATMA GANDHI

*C*onventions are a great way to see agency representatives and determine their interest in representing you as a model, gain insight into the business, and get feedback on your potential. Before you hand over your money to attend a convention, try to find out all you can about the company or sponsor. If the representative mentions the names of well-known agencies that will be attending, call some of them to find out if it is true.

Some of the top agencies in the world send representatives to conventions. However, as many of these professionals will tell you, while some conventions are hosted by reputable companies, others are a complete rip-off. It should be obvious if you are being charged thousands of dollars to attend. To give you an idea of what to expect at a reputable modeling convention, descriptions of three top-notch events follow.

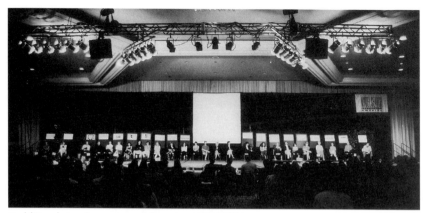

Model Search America agent panel discussion. MSA © 1999.

Model Search America

Model Search America (MSA) is a well-respected, ethical, and highly professional organization. F. David Mogull, president of Model Search America, is dedicated to providing a quality experience for attendees. His integrity is evident in the way he communicates with the models and the high caliber conventions he hosts. Mogull lets those interested in modeling know up front that the modeling industry is very competitive and that there are no guarantees.

At MSA, you have the chance to meet with representatives from New York, Miami, Chicago, Atlanta, Los Angeles, Europe, and Asia. Amazingly enough, the convention fee is very reasonable. In fact, you can see representatives from all of these markets for less money than it would cost you to purchase one super-saver airfare.

Representatives from the top modeling agencies might call back fifty models, twenty models, or none. It is important to understand that MSA is not a modeling competition or contest, and it is certainly not a beauty pageant. You will gain confidence in yourself, have a greater understanding of the modeling industry, and have fun. Attending a convention could be the first step in helping you decide if a modeling career is something you want to pursue. If you end up signing a contract with an agency, Model Search America receives a 5 percent scouting fee from the agency based on the earnings of the model, which is reasonable and customary.

MSA conventions are held in various cities across the United States, including Seattle; Washington, D.C.; Dallas; Atlanta; Kansas City; Rochester; Houston; New Orleans; Palm Springs; Cincinnati; Providence; Chicago; and Orlando. A partial list of the agencies that have been represented at MSA conventions in the past are:

- Agency Press, Tokyo
- Alexa Models
- Arlene Wilson
- Bailey's Model Management
- Bodyshop
- City Models
- Click Models
- Clipse Models
- Company Management
- Elite Model Management
- Empire
- Exposure
- FFT/Funny Face
- Generation
- Gilla Roos
- Halvorson Management
- ID Models
- Images
- IMG
- Jam

- Karin Models
- L'Agence
- LA Models
- Look Models
- Michele Pommier
- Millennium Models
- Mitchell Management
- Next
- Nova Models
- Nytro
- Page Parkes
- Prima Models
- Q Management
- Sage Models
- Satoru Models
- Talent Plus
- Taxi Models
- Traque Models
- Zoli Models

In addition to networking with agency representatives, participants of modeling conventions can also meet and learn from top professional models, hairstylists, makeup artists, actors, and casting directors. The following is a sample schedule from a weekend–long convention:

Saturday
- The International Modeling Business
- The Men's Modeling Business
- The Children's Modeling Business

- Commercial Print and Fashion Modeling
- Theater, Film, and the Television Industry
- How to Prepare for an Audition
- A Closer Look at TV Commercials
- All About Local Markets
- Seminars, Workshops, and Panel Discussions
- Hair and Makeup Trends
- Runway Guidance and Practice Sessions
- Autograph Sessions
- Saturday Night Party/Dance (alcohol-free)

Sunday

- Agency Introductions
- Agent Panel Discussion
- Individual Runway Presentation
- Individual Picture Review
- Callback Announcements
- Individual Interviews with Agencies

Note: "Callbacks" are the final portion of the convention, when announcements are made as to who has been chosen by each agency for possible representation. Those who receive callbacks will remain for individual interviews.

All models must bring photographs of themselves, which can be snapshots or Polaroids. If you have professional photographs or composite cards, bring them. You will need two different, current pictures to show the agents–a headshot and a full body shot–and one 3½" × 5" headshot for MSA's office use only. You should have five extra copies of your favorite picture in case an agent requests one. If you bring extra photographs and need some direction as to which ones to show the agents, on Saturday MSA staff can help you. On Saturday, dress casually, as you will not be seeing any agents. Sunday is an interview day, so you should dress in a stylish manner. Most importantly, be natural, be yourself, and have fun.

To attend a modeling convention through Model Search America, start with a free interview session. These are held all over the country throughout the year. To find out when Model Search America will be in your area, call the New York office at (212) 343–0100. Model Search America is located at 588 Broadway, Suite 711, New York, NY 10012. You can also find information on their Web site, *www.supermodel.com/aspire/msa.*

Modeling Association of America International, Inc.

The Modeling Association of America International, Inc. (MAAI), is the only nonprofit association that serves the modeling profession. This organization has been sponsoring conventions since 1960 and is managed by an advisory council and executive board of directors elected by the membership. MAAI's convention is held annually each April at the Waldorf–Astoria Hotel in New York City, inviting scouts and experts in the industry from all over the world to meet with the contestants. In addition to competitions in runway, photography, and television commercials, MAAI offers educational seminars and the chance to meet top agents. For more information, contact Ms. Betty Lane Gramlin, 250 Doyle Street, Orangeburg, SC 29115; (803) 534–9672. Or visit the MAAI Web site at *www.maai.org.*

New York Model Contracts

One talent scout told us that New York Model Contracts hosted one of the classiest conventions she ever attended. These conventions are not competitions, but are places where models can network with top agents, learn from professionals in workshops, and really get a feel for the business. Linda Bennett, president of New York Model Contracts, brings in the very best of agents and offers two rounds of callbacks. New York Model Contracts presents convention opportunities in approximately three hundred cities per year. Contact New York Model Contracts at 2424 Edenborn Avenue, Metairie, LA 70001; (504) 835–5654.

A Word about Rip-Off Conventions

Skip and I attempted to attend a convention scheduled in Los Angeles when we first started researching this book. Not only were we continuously put on hold, the company would not return our telephone calls and made excuse after excuse to keep us away from its convention. We became suspicious when we were not given any information about the convention, not even the cost to attend as a model. The company we are referring to has a very visible and impressive presence on the Internet.

Because of the strange way we were treated, we kept our eyes open as our research continued. It didn't take long to discover that quite a few models were very disappointed after attending this convention and felt they had been cheated. Most of them paid several thousand dollars to attend, only to be pitted against hundreds of other prospective models in a competition–type setting that provided networking opportunities with only a few agency representatives. For the amount of money these models paid to attend, they could have flown to New York with their families, stayed in a nice hotel, visited nearly every single major and minor agency, and probably still have had enough money left over for a Broadway show.

Conventions can be a great way to gain exposure, learn more about the business, and meet other models and professionals, but you should never have to pay thousands of dollars to attend. Some of the very best conventions, such as the ones mentioned earlier, offer very reasonable registration fees. Call and find out where they plan to be in the upcoming year. One of these conventions, we trust, is bound to be coming to a city near you.

CHAPTER NINETEEN

The Agencies

*"Many of life's failures are people who did not realize
how close they were to success when they gave up."*

THOMAS EDISON

*T*his book was written for all types of
people who want to work as models, no matter where they live. There
are modeling agencies in almost every state in the United States. While it
is not possible to list all of the agencies, especially in the smaller markets,
we decided to include a brief listing of the major U.S. markets, with an
emphasis on New York, and international markets, with an emphasis on
Paris.

The following information is offered for your consideration, investi-
gation, and judgment. By this we mean you must investigate each listing
for yourself. This industry experiences rapid, frequent change–not only
with fashion trends, but also with the management of the agencies themselves. Therefore, we do not endorse any of the agencies listed herein.
Before you begin your journey of finding an agency, please make sure
you have read chapters 6, 7, and 10.

If you plan to visit or submit photographs to some of the smaller, less-known agencies, contact them by telephone first to verify the address and if they are still in business. Since it is common for one agency to buy out another, relocate, or close its doors, some of the agency information listed here could have changed. When we began researching agencies, we prepared a mailing and sent it out to hundreds of agencies across the United States. We were amazed at how many envelopes came back marked "moved" or "not deliverable."

Open-call information and specific divisions within agencies are not listed; we suggest you contact the agencies directly and obtain this information. International agency information is provided in the major markets, but if you live in the United States, we stress the importance of working through a "mother" or home-based agency for international work.

Directories are available that focus entirely on providing agency information and are updated on an annual basis. Various modeling agency directories are published by Peter Glenn Publications, 42 West 38th Street, New York, NY 10018; (212) 869-2020. Also take a look at Model's Mart for reference materials and directories. Another great resource for finding out about agencies and general business practices within the industry is The Model's Guild, 265 West 14th Street, New York, NY 10011; (800) 864-4696 or (212) 675-4133. Although it is located in New York, The Model's Guild representatives can answer basic questions and provide information about agencies located in other major cities.

So whether you are seeking an agency in your hometown or in one of the major metropolitan areas, have fun in your search, and use your best judgment—and good luck!

United States

California

Click Model Management
9057 Nemo Street
North Hollywood, CA 90069
(310) 246-0800

Colleen Cler Agency for Kids
120 South Victory Boulevard #206
Burbank, CA 91502
(818) 841-7943
www.CCA4Kids.com

Colours
8344 West 3rd Street
Los Angeles, CA 90048
(213) 658-7072

Cunningham Agency
10635 Santa Monica Boulevard #130
Los Angeles, CA 90025
(310) 475-7573

Elite Model Management
345 North Maple Drive #397
Beverly Hills, CA 90210
www.elitemodel.com
(310) 274-9395

Ford Models Los Angeles
88826 Burton Way
Beverly Hills, CA 90011
(310) 276-8100
www.fordmodels.com

Industry
315 Pacific Avenue
San Francisco, CA 94111
(415) 733-5400

LA Models
8335 Sunset Boulevard
Los Angeles, CA 90069
(213) 656-9572
www.lamodels.com

Look
166 Geary Street #14900
San Francisco, CA 94108
(415) 781-2822

Next Model Management
8447 Wilshire Boulevard #301
Beverly Hills, CA 90211
(213) 782-0010

Nous Model Management
9157 Sunset Boulevard #212
Los Angeles, CA 90069
(310) 385-6900

Q Model Management
6100 Wilshire Boulevard, Suite 710
Los Angeles, CA 90048
(323) 692-1700
http://qmodels.com

Sirens Model Management
9455 Santa Monica Boulevard
Beverly Hills, CA 90210
(310) 246-1969

Specialty Models
8060 Melrose Avenue #225
Los Angeles, CA 90046
(213) 782-8999

Wilhelmina West, Inc.
8383 Wilshire Boulevard
Beverly Hills, CA 90211
(213) 655-0909 *(women–print)*
(213) 477-3112 *(men–print)*
www.wilhelmina.com

Florida

Click Modeling Agency
161 Ocean Drive
Miami Beach, FL 33139
(305) 674-9900

Elite Model Management
1200 Collins Avenue #207
Miami Beach, FL 33139
(305) 674-9500
www.elitemodel.com

Ford Models Florida
311 Lincoln Road, Suite 205
Miami, FL 33139
(305) 534-7200
www.fordmodels.com

Jump
1210 Washington Avenue #230
Miami, FL 33139
(305) 604-2558

Next Management
209 Ninth Street
Miami Beach, FL 33139
(305) 531-5100

Illinois

Aria Model & Talent Management
1017 West Washington, Suite 2C
Chicago, IL 60607
(312) 243-9400
ariamodel.com

Arlene Wilson Model Management
430 West Erie Street #210
Chicago, IL 60610
(312) 573-0200

Elite Model Management
58 West Huron Street
Chicago, IL 60610
(312) 943-3226
www.elitemodel.com

Emilia Lorence Models, Ltd.
619 North Wabash Avenue
Chicago, IL 60611
(312) 787-2033

ML International Modeling, Inc.
162 North Franklin Street
Chicago, IL 60606
(312) 849-9190

Models Unlimited
415 North LaSalle, Suite 202
Chicago, IL 60610
(312) 329-1001

Susanne Johnson Talent Agency, Ltd.
108 West Oak Street
Chicago, IL 60610
(312) 943–8315

New York

Aline Souliers Management
450 West 15th Street
New York, NY 10011
(212) 243–6565
(Women—fashion)

Click Models
129 West 27th Street
New York, NY 10001
(212) 206–1717
(Men and women—fashion)

Company Model Management
270 Lafayette Street, Suite 1400
New York, NY 10012
(212) 226–9190
(Women—fashion, print, runway)

Cunningham, Escott, Dipene & Assoc.
257 Park Avenue South, Suite 900
New York, NY 10010
(212) 477–3838
(Men, women, children, plus-size, petite)

Curves
524 Broadway, 4th Floor
New York, NY 10012
(212) 343–3661
(Women only—fit models, plus-size)

DNA Model Management
145 Hudson Street
New York, NY 10013
(212) 226–0080
(Men, women—fashion, catalog, print)

Elite Model Management
111 East 22nd Street
New York, NY 10010
(212) 529–9700 or (212) 475–1332
www.elitemodel.com
(Women only—fashion, runway)

Flaunt Models Management, Inc.
114 East 32nd Street, Suite 501
New York, NY 10016
(212) 679–9011
(Fashion, commercial, parts, plus-size)

Ford Models New York
142 Greene Street, 4th Floor
New York, NY 10012
(212) 219–6500
www.fordmodels.com
(Women, men, children, teens, plus-size, mature)

Funnyface Today, Inc.
151 East 31st Street
New York, NY 10016
(212) 686–4343
(Women, men, children—all categories)

Generations Model Management
18 West 20th Street
New York, NY 10011
(212) 727-7219
(Children)

Gilla Roos Ltd.
16 West 22nd Street, 3rd Floor
New York, NY 10010
(212) 727-7820
www.gillaroos.com
(Women, men, children—all categories)

ID Model Management
155 Spring Street, 3rd Floor
New York, NY 10012
(212) 941-5858
(Fashion)

Images Management
30 East 20th Street
New York, NY 10003
(212) 228-0300
(Men, women—fashion, print)

IMG Models
304 Park Avenue South
New York, NY 10010
(212) 253-8882
(Women—fashion, print)

Marilyn, Inc.
300 Park Avenue South
New York, NY 10010
(212) 260-6500
(Women—fashion)

Maxx Men
30 East 20th Street
New York, NY 10003
(212) 228-0278
(Men only)

Mega Models
594 Broadway #507
New York, NY 10012-3234
(212) 334-5800
(Women, children)

Next Management
23 Watts Street
New York, NY 10013
(212) 925-5100
(Women, men)

Parts Models
P.O. Box 7529
FDR Station
New York, NY 10150
(212) 744-6129
(Parts models—send professional photos/
composites only)

Paulines
379 West Broadway
New York, NY 10012
(212) 941–6000
(Women only)

Q Model Management
180 Varick Street, Floor 13
New York, NY 10014
(212) 807–6777
http://qmodels.com

R&L Model Management
645 5th Avenue
New York, NY 10022
(212) 935–2300
www.blackwood-steele.com

Rachel's Totz N Teenz
134 West 29th Street
New York, NY 10001
(212) 967–3167
(Children—all categories)

Wilhelmina International, Ltd.
300 Park Avenue South
New York, NY 10010
(212) 473–0700
www.wilhelmina.com
(Women, men—fashion, print, plus-size)

Women Model Management
107 Greene Street
New York, NY 10012
(212) 334–7480
(Women—catalog, editorial)

Zoli Model Management
3 West 18th Street
New York, NY 10011
(212) 242–5959
(Women, men—all categories)

Texas

Elan Model & Talent Management
4215 McEwen Road
Dallas, TX 75244
(214) 239–2398

Kim Dawson
1643 Apparel Mart
Dallas, TX 75258
(214) 638–2414

Model's Rep
3303 Lee Parkway
Dallas, TX 75219
(214) 526–4434

International

Australia

Camerons
163 Broughan Street
Sydney, NSW 2011
612-358-6433

Chadwicks
32A Oxford Street, 2nd Floor
Sydney, NSW 2010
612-332-4177

Chic Model Management
155 New South Head Road
Edge Cliff, NSW 2027
612-328-6900

Priscilla's
185 Elizabeth Street
Sydney, NSW 2000
612-261-1512

Vivien's
43 Bay Street, 1st Floor
Double Bay
Sydney, NSW 2028
612-326-2700

Brazil

Elite Model Management
Rue Sampaio Vidal 1096
São Paolo, SP 01443
55-11-210-4355
www.elitemodel.com

Ford Models Brazil
Rue Bento de Andrade 421
Jardim Paulista
CEP 04503-011
55-11-884-5920
www.fordmodels.com.br

Taxi
Av. Sao Gabriel 564
São Paolo, SP 01435
55-11-887-9755

Canada

Alexander Model
610 1155 West Georgia
Vancouver, BC V6E 3H4
604-658-1043

Charles Stuart
1008 Homer
Vancouver, BC V6B 3H6
604-683-2267

Christie's Model & Talent
    Management
22 Arbour Crest Road Northwest
Calgary, Alberta T3G 4J9
403-651-3389

Folio, Inc.
373 Place D'Youville 301
Montreal, Quebec H2Y 2B7
514-288-8080

Ford Models Canada
385 Adelaide Street West
Toronto, Ontario M5V 1S4
416-362-9208
www.fordmodels.com

International Top Models
119 Spadina Avenue
Toronto, Ontario M5V 2L1
416-979-9995

Select Model Management, Ltd.
10247 124th Street
Edmonton, Alberta T5N 1P8
780-482-2828

Sub Zero Management
624 Richmond Street West
Toronto, Ontario M5V 3C2
416-203-6522

Sutherland Models
174 Spadina #100
Toronto, Ontario M5T 2C2
416-703-7070

Thomas Models
9-1035 Richards Street
Vancouver, BC V6B 3E4
604-683-1262

China

Galaxy International Model Management *(formerly New Silk Road)*
2/F, No. 3 Dofang Road
Dongsanhuan Beilu, Beijing 100027
10-6462-8134

England

Assassin Management Ltd.
2 Marshall Street
London W1V 1LQ
171-534-5400

Bookings
6 Pembridge Studios
27A Pembridge Villas
London W11 3EP
171-221-2603

Boss
33 Marshall Street
London W1V 1LL
171-439-2444

Crawfords
2 Conduit Street
London W1R 9TG
171-629-6464

Elite Premier Model Agency
40–42 Parker Street
London WC2B 5PQ
171-333-0888

Gavin Models
11 Old Burlington Street
London W1X 1LA
171-629-5231

Image
81 Wimpole Street
London W1M 7DB
171-935-9021

IMG
13-16 Jacob Well Mews
George Street
London W1H 5PD
171-486-8011

Model Plan
Harbour Yard
Chelsea Harbour
Unit 4, 3rd Floor
London SW10 OXD
171-351-3244

Models One
Omega House
471 Kings Road
London SW10 0LU
171-351-1195

Mystique Model Management, Ltd.
International House
8 Wendell Road
London W12 9RT
181-749-7771

Nev's
Regal House
198 Kings Road
London SW3 SXP
171-352-4886

Norrie Carr Modeling Agency
30 Fryent Way
London NW9 9SB
181-204-2241

Respect Model Agency
Unit 202
The Custard Factory
Gibb Street
Birmingham B4AA
0121-693-1223

Select Model Agency
43 King Street
London WC2
171-470-5222

Storm
45 Marloes Road
London W8 6LA
171-938-4033

Top Models
21-25 Goldhawk Road, 3rd Floor
London W12 8QQ
181-743-0640

Truly Scrumptious
Holborn Studios
10 Black Hill
London EC1R 5EN
171-278-4311

Ugly
Tigris House
256 Edgeware Road
London W2 1DS
171-402-5564

France

AAC
10, avenue George V
75008 Paris
Tél. (01) 47 23 01 66
Fax. (01) 53 67 79 31
(Men, women)

Allix
80, rue Vaneau
75007 Paris
Tél. (01) 42 84 03 03
Fax. (01) 45 44 18 94
(Children)

Bananas Mambo
9, rue Duphot
75001 Paris
Tél. (01) 40 20 02 03
Fax. (01) 40 20 41 20
(Men)

Beauties/V.O. Models
22, rue Caumartin
75009 Paris
Tél. (01) 47 42 51 79
Fax. (01) 47 42 01 51
(Women, men)
• *V.O. is the advertising section of Beauties:*
Tél. (01) 42 66 31 38
Fax. (01) 42 66 33 81

Bout'chou
22, rue Brey
75017 Paris
Tél. (01) 45 72 34 35
Fax. (01) 45 72 41 06
(Children)

City Models
21, rue Jean Mermoz
75008 Paris
Tél. (01) 53 93 33 33
Fax. (01) 53 93 33 34
(Women)

Clapboard International
2, rue Pierre Demours
75017 Paris
Tél. (01) 45 72 17 55
Fax. (01) 45 72 21 71
(Women, men—specializes in advertising)

Click Model Management
27, rue Vernet–2nd étage
75008 Paris
Tél. (01) 47 23 44 00
Fax. (01) 47 20 31 15
(Men, women)

Coccinelle
28, rue de Trévise
75009 Paris
Tél. (01) 42 46 55 00
Fax. (01) 42 46 07 94
(Men, women, children—specializes in
advertising)

Company Management
48, rue Sainte-Anne
75002 Paris
Tél. (01) 40 20 42 20
Fax. (01) 40 20 42 21
(Women, men—specializes in details,
sportsmen, ethnics, seniors)

Crystal Model Agency
9, rue Duphot
75001 Paris
Tél. (01) 42 61 98 98
Fax. (01) 42 61 90 47
(Women)

Cute Models
28, rue Cardinet
75017 Paris
Tél. (01) 44 40 45 45
Fax. (01) 44 40 45 44
(Children)

Cyrano/Roxane
25, rue de Ponthieu
75008 Paris
Tél. (01) 44 95 84 50
Fax. (01) 44 95 84 69
(Men, women—specializes in advertising)

D.I.
17, rue des Petits Champs
75001 Paris
Tél. (01) 42 97 54 91 / 42 97 01 42
Fax. (01) 40 20 98 49
(Men, children—specializes in advertising)

Dynamite
34, rue de Laborde
75008 Paris
Tél. (01) 42 94 89 89
Fax. (01) 42 94 89 00
(Men, children—specializes in advertising)

Elite Model Management
8, bis, rue Lecuirot
75008 Paris
Tél. (01) 40 44 32 22
Fax. (01) 40 44 32 80
www.elitemodel.com
(Women, minimum age sixteen. Appoint-
ments necessary.)

F.A.M. International
30, bd Vital–Bouhot
92200 Neuilly sur Seine
Tél. (01) 41 92 06 50
Fax. (01) 46 37 45 50
(Women)

Figures Libres
14, bis, rue Marbeuf
75008 Paris
Tél. (01) 49 52 08 00
Fax. (01) 47 20 96 20
(Men and women)

Ford Models Europe/Ford Line
9, rue Scribe
75009 Paris
Tél. (01) 53 05 25 25
Fax. (01) 53 05 25 26
www.fordmodels.com
(Women)

Frimousse
8, rue de Ponthieu
75008 Paris
Tél. (01) 53 75 40 40
Fax. (01) 53 75 40 41
(Children)

Glady's' Fashion
4, avenue Verguin
69006 Lyon
Tél. (04) 78 94 07 80
Fax. (04) 78 89 10 92
(Men, women)

H.O.H./Profil by Success
64, rue Rambuteau
75003 Paris
Tél. (01) 40 29 04 04
Fax. (01) 42 78 23 88
(Men, women)

Idole Model Management
3, rue du Cirque
75008 Paris
Tél. (01) 53 96 06 00
Fax. (01) 53 96 06 01
(Women)

International Management Group
2, rue Dufrenoy
75116 Paris
Tél. (01) 45 03 85 00
Fax. (01) 45 03 85 01
(Men, women; models, artists, and athletes)

Karin Models/Men of Karin
9, avenue Hoche
75008 Paris
Tél. (01) 45 63 08 23
Fax. (01) 45 63 58 18
(Men, women)
• Men of Karin is the men's section:
Tél. (01) 45 63 33 69
Fax. (01) 45 63 17 71

La Recre
11, rue Jacques Coeur
75004 Paris
Tél. (01) 42 78 48 22
Fax. (01) 42 71 88 93
(Children)

Les Moins de 20 Ans
11, rue de Navarrin
75009 Paris
Tél. (01) 42 82 12 12
Fax. (01) 42 82 72 02
(Children, juniors—same group as Karin)

Madison Models
4, avenue Hoche
75008 Paris
Tél. (01) 44 29 26 36
Fax. (01) 47 63 44 04
(Women—specializes in photography and
advertising)

Marilyn Agency/MGM/Mar. Sports
4, rue de la Paix
75002 Paris
Tél. (01) 53 29 53 53
Fax. (01) 53 29 53 00
(Men, women, children)
• Men's section:
Tél. (01) 53 29 53 39
Fax. (01) 53 29 53 02
• Sportsmen and celebrities section:
Tél. (01) 53 29 53 49
Fax. (01) 53 29 53 30

MAS
3, rue du Colonel Moll
75017 Paris
Tél. (01) 40 68 71 30
Fax. (01) 45 72 46 62
(Women, men)

Media Acteurs, Jean-Luc Darler
34, rue Vivienne
75002 Paris
Tél. (01) 44 82 79 80
Fax. (01) 44 88 20 89
(Men, children—specializes in advertising)

Metropolitan/PHM/Metropub
7, bd des Capucines
75002 Paris
Tél. (01) 42 66 52 85
Fax. (01) 42 66 48 75
(Women, men—three departments: women,
men, and advertising)

Models, Evelyne Lichardy, PDG
Hôtel de Retz
75003 Paris
Tél. (01) 40 29 47 47
Fax. (01) 40 29 47 46
(Women)

Nathalie
10, rue Daubigny
75017 Paris
Tél. (01) 44 29 07 10
Fax. (01) 44 29 07 11
(Women)

Next Management
188, rue de Rivoli
75001 Paris
Tél. (01) 53 45 13 00
Fax. (01) 53 45 13 01
(Men, women)

Ovation
17, rue André del Sarte
75018 Paris
Tél. (01) 42 59 14 00
Fax. (01) 42 59 14 15
(Women, men—specializes in advertising)

Partners Model Management
7, avenue de Villiers
75017 Paris
Tél. (01) 47 54 91 00
Fax. (01) 47 54 92 00
(Women)

People/Funny Faces
39, rue Ste Croix de la Bretonnerie
75004 Paris
Tél. (01) 40 29 99 00
Fax. (01) 40 29 90 81
(Women, men)

Perfect Models
B.P. 417
62225 Calais Cedex
Tél. (03) 21 97 53 84
Fax. (03) 21 97 81 55
(Women, men, children; also has a branch in Seoul, Korea)

PH One/Absolu/Public
50, rue Etienne Marcel
75002 Paris
Tél. (01) 44 76 58 70
Fax. (01) 44 76 58 71
(Men, women—has three departments: PH One for men; Absolu for women; and Public for advertising)

Rebecca
33, rue du Petit Musc
75004 Paris
Tél. (01) 44 61 84 20
Fax. (01) 44 61 84 21
(Men, children)

Sindy Bop
12, rue du Général Percin
33400 Talence
Tél. (05) 56 80 18 45
Fax. (05) 56 80 18 45
(Men, women, children)

Success/Success Kids
64, rue Rambuteau
75003 Paris
Tél. (01) 42 78 69 69
Fax. (01) 42 78 80 02
(Men, children)
• Success Kids:
Tél. (01) 42 78 87 87

Talent Fashion
320, rue Saint-Honoré
69, rue d'Hauteville
75010 Paris
Tél. (01) 42 46 83 72
(Women—same group as You Models
Management)

Tally Ho/Ever and Ever
104, rue de la Faisanderie
75116 Paris
Tél. (01) 42.60.01.36
Fax. (01) 49.26.08.73
(Women)

Viva!
15, rue Duphot
75001 Paris
Tél. (01) 44 55 12 60
Fax. (01) 44 55 12 62
(Women—same group as Elite)

Germany

Berlin Models
Rosenthalerstrasse 3
1054 Berlin
2805–126

D'Selection
Benratherstrasse 6A
4000 Dusseldorf
02-11-84555

E-Models
Bastionstrasse 27
4000 Dusseldorf 1
02-11-132475

Frankfurt One
Hamburger Allee 45, 60486
69-975-875-0

Heide Themlitz
Ohmstrasse 5
8000 Munich 40
089-397018

Jacqueline's
Tubingerstrasse 83A
7000 Stuttgart 1
0711-603040

Klages Models
Adalbertstrasse 108
8000 Munich 40
089-2710271

Louisa Models
Ebersberger Strasse 9
8000 Munich 80
089-921096-20

Mega
Wexstrasse 26
D-2000 Hamburg 36
040-343009

Model Management
Hartungstrasse 5
2000 Hamburg 5
040-440555

Model Pool
Rathausufer 23
4000 Dusseldorf 1
02-11-132171

Model Team
Schluterstrasse 60
2 Hamburg 13
040-4141037

Munich Models
Karl Theodorestrasse 18A
8000 Munich 40
089-341336

Network
Rothenbaumchausse 83
2000 Hamburg 13
040-441451

Promod
Bieberstrasse 9
2000 Hamburg 13
040-443399

Talents
Muhlenkamp 31
2000 Hamburg 60
040-271047

Italy

Casting
Via Cavour 31
50129 Firenze
055-238-1348

Elite Model Management
Via San Vittore 40
20123 Milano
481-4704
www.elitemodel.com

Eye for I
Via Guerrazzi 1
20145 Milano
2-345471

Flash
Via Mantova 11
20135 Milano
55-187277

Italy Model Agency
Piazza Sicilia 6
20146 Milano
4801-2828

Look Now
Via Forcella 13
20144 Milano
8940-0165

Model Plan
Via Revere 8
20123 Milano
4800-2712

My Models
Via A. Manuzio 17
20124 Milano
657-0241

Theluxe Models
Via Tortona 15
20144 Milano
2-581-7781

Want Models
Via Borgonuovo 10
20121 Milano
2-290-6631

Japan

Chic
3-52-5 Sendegaya
Shibuya-Ku Tokyo 151
33-478-5867

Cinq-Deux-Un
#508 9-6-28 Alaska
Minato-Ku Tokyo 107
33-402-8445

Elite Folio
3F, 3-16-15 Roppongi
Minato-Ku Tokyo 106
33-587-0200

Zem Models
Osaka Ekimae No. 2
Bldg. 2F, 1-2-2
Umeda Kita-ku 530
6-341-5252

Scotland

Model Team Scotland
166 Buchanan Street
Glasgow G1 2LW
041-332-3951

CHAPTER TWENTY

Resources

*"Your work is to discover your work, and then
with all your heart, to give yourself to it."*

BUDDHA

*I*n the ever-changing world of fash-
ion, some of the agency or Web site information listed in this chapter
could change by the time this book is printed. There are a great many
resources listed here, but we urge you to always use your good judgment
as to the legitimacy of any references presented here. Have fun exploring!

Books

General Modeling

Anderson Boyd, Marie. *Model: The Complete Guide for Men and Women.* New York:
Peter Glen Publications, 1997. This is an absolutely beautiful book, filled with
photos, illustrations, and practical information about modeling.

Esch, Natasha; Rebecca Gayheart; and Christine Walker. *The Wilhelmina Guide to
Modeling.* New York: Fireside, 1996.

Givhan, Robin. Photographs by Lucien Perkins. *Runway Madness*. San Francisco: Chronicle Books, 1998.

Matheson, Eve. *The Modeling Handbook: The Complete Guide to Breaking into Local, Regional, and International Modeling*. New York: Peter Glenn Publications, 1999. This book is in its fourth edition, and for good reason: It extensively covers what it is like to work in the modeling profession, including information regarding international as well as domestic modeling.

Morris, Sandra. *Catwalk: Inside the World of the Supermodels*. New York: Universe Publishing, 1996.

———. *The Model Manual: Everything You Need to Know about Modeling*. London: George Weidenfeld and Nicolson Ltd, 1997.

Preston, Karl. *Modelmania: The Working Model's Manual*. Marina Del Rey, CA: Dog Gone Books, 1998. Karl is a top male model based out of southern California who offers a wealth of experience regarding all aspects of the business.

Rose, Yvonne; Tony Rose; Natalie Robinson (illustrator); and Wayne Summerlin (photographer). *Is Modeling for You? The Handbook and Guide for the Young Aspiring Black Model*. Phoenix: Amber Books, 1997.

Rubinstein, Donna, and Jennifer Kingston Bloom. *The Modeling Life: The One (and Only) Book that Gives You the Inside Story of What the Business Is Like and How You Can Make It*. New York: Perigee, 1998.

Summers, Barbara. *Skin Deep: Inside the World of Black Fashion Models*. New York: Amistad Press, 1999. This book covers the history of beautiful Black women who have made an impact on the world of style and provides insight from the Black model's perspective.

Directories

International Directory of Model and Talent Agencies & Schools. New York: Peter Glenn Publications, 1999. Contains more than 2,500 listings of schools, agencies, associations, conventions, pageants, managers, and casting directors. You can purchase this book directly through the publisher: 42 West 38th Street, New York, NY 10018; (212) 869–2020.

Makeup

Aucoin, Kevyn. *Making Faces*. New York: Little Brown & Co., 1997. A truly amazing book—offering 60 instructional watercolor sketches. This book is a work of art, featuring the world's most renowned makeup artists' secrets display in 240 color photos. Kevyn Aucoin is the makeup artist behind many magazine covers and is a recipient of the Council of Fashion Designers of America (CFDA) Award for makeup artistry. Kevyn has also written a book called *Making Faces*, which details even more makeup techniques and skin–care information.

Begoun, Paula, and Sigrid Asmus. *Don't Go to the Cosmetics Counter Without Me: An Eye-Opening Guide to Brand-Name Cosmetics.* Seattle, WA: Beginning Press, 1998.

Brown, Bobbi, and Annemarie Iverson. *Bobbi Brown Beauty: The Ultimate Beauty Resource.* New York: Harper Perennial Library, 1998. Written by a well-known, professional makeup artist, this book is filled with illustrations and information on makeup application.

Fine, Sam, and Julia Chance. *Fine Beauty: Beauty Basics and Beyond for African-American Women.* New York: Putnam Publishing Group, 1998. This beautifully illustrated book offers tips and step-by-step instructions on makeup application for African-American women.

Walker, Andre, and Teresa Wiltz. *Andre Talks Hair.* New York: Simon & Schuster, 1997. This book is filled with information about hair care—from figuring out your hair type to taking care of your hair to hair coloring—for all types of women. By the way, Andre Walker is Oprah's personal hairstylist.

Wells, Reggie, and Theresa Foy Digeronimo. *Face Painting: African-American Beauty Techniques from an Emmy Award–Winning Makeup Artist.* New York: Henry Holt and Company, Inc., 1998.

Fashion

Cho, Emily, and Neila Fisher. *Instant Style: 500 Professional Tips on Fashion, Beauty, and Attitude.* New York: Harper Collins, 1996.

Acting

Alterman, Glenn. *Promoting Your Acting Career.* New York: Allworth Press, 1998. Provides voluminous information on the business side of an acting career.

Self Improvement and Beauty

Emme, and Daniel Paisner. *True Beauty: Positive Attitudes and Practical Tips from the World's Leading Plus-Size Model.* New York: Perigee, 1998. A beautiful book on overcoming negative body images and developing a positive self–image.

Other

Gross, Michael. *Model: The Ugly Business of Beautiful Women.* New York: William Morrow and Company, Inc., 1996. One of the most comprehensive and revealing books on the modeling industry that you will find. Contains extensive historical information along with a discussion of the less desirable aspects of the business. The updated paperback version contains insight on the decline of the supermodel.

Hollenbeck, Cliff. *Swimsuit Model Photography.* New York: Amherst Media, 1997.

Pegram, Billy. *Fashion Model Photography: Professional Techniques and Images.* New York: Amherst Media, 1999. Covers all aspects of fashion-model photography and gives the professional model a working knowledge of what takes place on the other side of the camera.

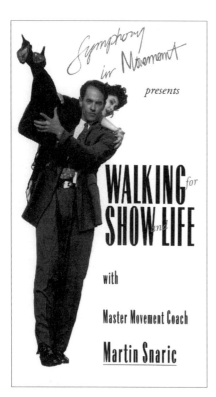

Videos

The Art of Modeling, hosted by Kristen Jensen, is a great video that shows you what the world of modeling is like. It is beautiful, well put together, informative, and entertaining. You can obtain a copy through Model's Mart, or by contacting Ivy Hill Productions at (888) ART-1011. See also *www.amazon.com/exec/ obidos/ASIN/6305020914/webcraftcomput05/002- 8310076-2885849.*

Walking for Show and Life, by world-renowned walking coach Martin Snaric. To purchase a copy, contact Symphony in Movement, 41–22 42nd Street, Suite 1G, Long Island City, NY 11104.*www.SymphonyInMovement.com/index4. html.*

Working the Runway is a video for the beginning model, by Erin Ashley. You can purchase this video by mail. Send $14.95 in check or money order, plus $5 shipping and handling to the Models Connection, 32 Karen Place, Newbury Park, CA 91320. Allow 3–6 weeks for delivery.

Makeup Products/Lessons

Makeup For Ever Professional, SoHo Boutique, 409 West Broadway, New York, NY; (212) 941–9337; fax (212) 941–9338. If you are in New York, try to visit this boutique. This is a fantastic place to have a professional makeup lesson and try these products. Expect to pay around $50 to $60 for a makeup lesson.

Modeling Supplies and Books

Models Mart, 42 West 38th Street, New York, NY 10018; (212) 944–0638; fax (212) 869–3287; *www.models-mart.com.* Models Mart carries books, directories, videos, portfolios–everything the model needs to get started. Most of the books listed in this chapter can be purchased there.

Peter Glenn Publications, 42 West 38th Street, Suite 802, New York, NY 10018; (212) 869–2020; *http://peterglennpublications.com*

Composite Cards and Digital Services

DICE, 101 Fifth Avenue, Sixth Floor, New York, NY 10003; (212) 255–2711

MG Prints, 150 Varick Street, Third Floor, New York, NY 10013; (212) 337–3400

Modern Postcard, 1675 Faraday Avenue, Carlsbad, CA 92008; (800) 959–8365; (760) 431–1939 (fax); *http://modernpostcard.com*

Web Sites

Our Favorites

There are so many fantastic fashion–modeling Web sites available that it will take you weeks to fully explore them all. We've highlighted a few of our favorites to help you get started in your research. Have fun!

http://advocacy-net.com/modelmks.htm. This is one of the best Web sites with which to start. It provides a long listing of hundreds of modeling–related Web sites for you to investigate. Be patient, because it takes time to download all these sites!

http://modelnetwork.com. A great site devoted to providing models with all the information needed to get started. You will find agency information, facts about some of your favorite models, advice on modeling, and a listing of great resource material.

http://modelnews.com. Bookmark this site, because you will refer back to it again and again. It offers a free modeling evaluation, tips for beginning models, a model-of-the-month contest, a scam watch, and information on agencies, supermodels, hair, makeup, and skin care.

www.models-mart.com. This is a fantastic Web site that offers modeling-related supplies and resources by mail order. This site has a newsletter that provides up-to-date information on new books, agencies, and events. Models Mart has been in business for more than twenty-eight years.

http://go-international.com. Go International Model Management's Web site is perfect for anyone seeking information about starting a modeling career. It's listed as a favorite for several reasons: Mona Overton, the owner of the agency, has been in the business for more than thirty years. She and her partner, Kathy Robertson, have a strong Internet presence and are very helpful to new models. Also, they don't care where you live. Mona and Kathy will take a look at your photographs, and if they believe they'll be able to find you work, you don't have to relocate. Since they book models in various international markets, you might be expected to travel to Japan, Europe, or who knows where for modeling opportunities. They are also instrumental in helping models become established with top modeling agencies.

Newsgroups and Forums

Le Forum d'Annonces (French site): *http://disc.server.com/Indices/56393.html*

Hypermode Model Forum: *http://models.com/meta/forum/*

New Models: *www.newmodels.com/chat*

New York Models and Photographers Forum: *www.senac.com/forums/1406/*

The Nine Models International: *www.ninemodels.com*

The Talent Alliance (THETA): *http://thetalentalliance.com/forums/*

http://Duori.com/fashionforum/index.html

http://Modelforum.com/wwwboard/index.html

http://www.vangargoyle.com/visitors/index.html

Cosmetics

Beautynet: *www.beautynet.com*

Clinique: *http://clinique.com*

Cosmetic Index–Source and Resources for the Cosmetic Industry: *www.cosmeticindex.com/*

Face Art: *www.faceart.com*

Heather Kleinman's Cosmetic Connection: *http://cosmeticconnection.com*

Makeup Artist Magazine: *http://makeupmag.com/home.htm*

Modeling Contests

Ford Model Agency's Supermodel of the Year contest. (See *www.fordmodels.com* for more information.)

Elite Model Management's Elite Model Look contest. (See *www.elitemodels.com.sg/home/home.html* for more information.)

L.A. Model's L.A. Look of the Year contest. (See *http://lamodels.com.*)

Wilhelmina's plus–size modeling contest, cosponsored with *Mode* Magazine.

Consumer Protection

Better Business Bureau: *http://newyork.bbb.org/library/publications/tt1903.html#top; www.bbbsouthland.org/topic116.html; www.bbb.org/library/model.html*

Consumer and Consumer Protection Links: *www.onlinenews.net/consumer.html*

The Consumer Law Page: *http://consumerlawpage.com*

Federal Trade Commission Consumer Protection: *www.ftc.gov/ftc/consumer.htm*

Federal Trade Commission information for models: *www.ftc.gov/bcp/conline/pubs/services/model.htm*

Fashion

Fashion Alley: A Place Where Fashion, Trends, and Style Resides: *www.fashionalley.net*

The Fashion House: *www.valuenetwork.com/valu-net/fashion.htm*

Fashion Live (See fashion shows from Paris, Milan, New York): *www.worldmedia.fr/fashion/indexva.html*

Fashion Net–Your Guide to Fashion on the Net: *http://fashion.net/*

Fashion Planet: *www.fashion-planet.com/*

First View: *www.firstview.com/*

La Mode Francaise: *www.lamodefrancaise.tm.fr/*

Lumiére: *www.lumiere.com/*

New York Style: *www.nystyle.com/*

Place De Mode: *www.placedemode.com/*

Modeling Information

America Models Network: *http://americamodels.com*

Amerimall.com's Model Central: *http://amerimall.com/model/index.html*

Asian Model.Net: *http://asianmodel.net*

BluFire Model Registry: *http://sapphire.com/blufire/*

Eastman Agency Inc.: *http://eastmanmodel-film.com*

Fashion Models: On the Net 500 Sites: *http://whatsonthe.net/modelmks.htm*

Fashion Showroom: *http://fashionshowroom.com*

Global Model Registry: *www.galaxymall.com/Model/travel.html*

How To Model.com: *http://howtomodel.com*

International Modeling Market Information: *www.galaxymall.com/Model/travel.html*

International Models.com: *www.internationalmodels.com*

The Looks: *www.thelooks.com*

Models.com: *http://models.com*

Models Mart: *http://models-mart.com*

Model Network: *http://modelnetwork.com*

Model News.com: *http://modelnews.com*

Model Promote: *www.modelpromote.com*

Model Scout, Inc.: *http://modelscout.com*

Models Online: *http://models-online.com*

Models Page: *http://modelspage.com*

Model Source: *http://modelsource.com*

New Wave Images: *http://newwaveimages.com*

New Faces Talent Entertainment Industry Portfolios: *www.newfaces.com*

The Nine Models International: *www.ninemodels.com*

Pro–Model World Wide: *http://pro-model.com*

Top Models International Model Management: *www.topmodels.com.au*

Tracey International Spokes–model: *www.spokesmodel.com*

'Web Models: *www.webmodels.com*

Organizations

The Modelling Association of Canada: *http://models-online.com/gateway/news/maoc/ maoc.html*. This nonprofit organization promotes and maintains high standards in the modeling business.

The Model's Guild: *themodelsguild.org*. A great resource to utilize for finding out about agencies and general business practices within the industry is The Model's Guild, located at 265 West 14th Street, New York, NY 10011. Their telephone numbers are (800) 864–4696 and (212) 675–4133. Although the Guild is located in New York City, they will answer any questions you might have and give you information about agencies located in the major cities.

International Freelance Models Organisation (IFMO), Australia: *www.ifmo.com.au*

Models on the Web: Our Favorite Sites

http://carolalt.net
http://firstsupermodel.com
http://kathyireland.com
http://web-search.com/photo2.html#mod
http://zoy.com
www.fashion.tripnet.se/models.htm
www.frederique.com
www.supermodel.com

Magazines

Clique: www.cyberus.ca/~clique
E-News Electronic Newsstand (links to hundreds of magazines): *www.enews.com*
Tear Sheet magazine: *http://modelnetwork.com/tearsheet*
Teen magazine: *http://teenmag.com*
Vogue: http://vogue.co.uk
Women's Wear Daily: www.wwd.com/

Education

http://fashioncollege.com. Fashion Careers of California College Online is a private post–secondary business school for those seeking careers in the fashion industry. Telephone: (888) FCC–C999.

http://makeupschool.com. The Los Angeles School of Makeup offers professional courses in fashion makeup as well as special effects. The school is located at 10153 Riverside Drive, Toluca Lake, CA 91602. Phone: (818) 752–4276.

Agencies and Model Management Companies

Aria Model and Talent: *www.ariamodel.com*

Arlene Wilson Management: *http://arlenewilson.com*

Bailey's Model Management: *http://cbmodels.com*

Boston Models: *http://bostonmodelo.com*

CB Group Talent Management: *http://cbgroup.com*

Classic Model and Talent Management: *www.rivint.com/classic*

Concept Model Management, Inc.: *http://conceptmodels.com*

Contempo Models (Mexico City): *www.contempomodels.com*

Directions USA: *www.electricpaving.com/directions/*

Diva Models (Singapore): *http://divamodels.com.sg*

Donna Baldwin Talent, Inc.: *www.donnabaldwin.com*

Dreams International Model & Casting Agency: *www.dreamsagency.com*

Dynasty Models & Talent Inc.: *www.dynastymodels.com*

E Model Management: *http://emodelmanagement.com*

Eastern Models (Poland): *www.ikard.waw.pl/em/index.html*

Eastman Agency: *http://eastmanmodel-film.com*

Elite Model Management: *www.elitemodel.com*

Empire Model Management: *http://empirela.com*

The Erickson Agency: *http://ericksonagency.com*

Excel Talent (Division of Go International): *http://exceltalent.com*

Fameagency (conventions/trade shows/fashion): *http://fameagency.com*

Firestone Modeling and Talent Agency: *http://firestonemodeling.com*

Flair Modeling and Talent: *www.flairmodeling.com*

Ford Model Management, Inc.: *www.fordmodels.com*

Front Agency (Sweden): *www.algonet.se/front/*

Go International Model Management: *http://go-international.com*

Grant Models International: *http://grantmodels.com*

Halvorson Model Management: *http://models-online.com/Halvorson*

ICE Model Talent Management (Toronto): *http://icemodels.com*

J. Ballard Model and Talent Management: *http://jballard.com*

L.A. Models: *http://lamodels.com*

Look Model Management: *http://lookmodel.com*

MAG Models: *www.cadvision.com/magmod/*

Model Guide (Karim Ramzi): *www.modelguide.net*

Model Management International: *http://modelmgmt.com*

Models East: *http://modelseast.com*

Otto Model Management: *www.ottomodels.com*

Paparazzi Model Management (Finland): *http://paparazzi.fi/*

Paradox Model and Talent Management (Australia): *http://paradoxm.com.au/*

Q Model Management: *http://qmodels.com*

R & L Model Management: *http://blackwood-steele.com*

Rores Modeling Agency (Poland): *www.mediagalleries.com/rores*

Spirit Model Management: *http://spiritmodels.com*

Starmaker Models, Talent & Casting: *www.starsusa.com*

Stars: *http://starsagency.com*

TAC Model & Talent Management: *www.modeling.cc*

Talent Source: *http://talentsource.com*

Talent Trek Agency: *http://talentrek.com*

Taxi Model Management: *http://taximodels.com*

Tyler Models: *http://models-online.com/Tyler/*

Wilhelmina International, Ltd.: *www.wilhelmina.com*

World Model Management: *http://worldmodelmgmt.com*

Other Information

American Federation of Television and Radio Artists (AFTRA): *www.aftra.com/home.html*

Digicomps™: *http://modelnetwork.com/services/digicomp.html*

Screen Actors Guild (SAG): *http://sag.com*

Spokesmodel International, LLC: *www.spokesmodel.com*

Photographers

Global Photographer Search: *http://photographers.com*

MJP Artists is owned by molly J Peterson, who after twenty-five years in the arena of education, has embarked on a career in the creative fields of photography and fashion. Molly uses the latest technology to get her talent seen and is adept at personal contact for matching talent to specific client needs. Matching client to artist is of paramount importance. MJP is located at 8033 Sunset Boulevard, Suite 243, Los Angeles, CA 90046. E-mail can be sent to *mjpart@ pacbell.com.*

Photo Resource magazine: *www.photoresource.com*

Photographers of Note: *www.execpc.com/~torrey/notefoto.html*

Contributing Photographers and Artists

Photographers

Andrei—www.andreiphoto.com

Andrei began shooting at the age of five in Minsk, Belarus, under the guidance of his grandfather. In 1980, he emigrated to the United States, where he honed his photographic talents at Columbia College in Chicago, the Minneapolis College of Art & Design, and finally the School of Communication Arts.

While working at Studio210 of Minneapolis in collaboration with Mykl Randle, a former assistant to the legendary Herb Ritts, Andrei quickly gained a reputation for highly stylized work and his use of unique theatrical lighting, optical special effects, and custom-developed film processing techniques, all accomplished without resorting to computer enhancement. Now, equipped with a state-of-the-art digital image manipulation lab, he continues to push the limits of modern photography.

Chosen by the Luen Thai Corporation of Hong Kong (partner to such fashion giants as Tommy Hilfiger, DKNY, Liz Claiborne, Perry Ellis, Nautica, Nordstrom, Macy's, and Ralph Lauren) to provide the imagery which helped launch J18, a fashion retail chain now franchised throughout Asia, Andrei has served a world-wide list of clients, including: Condé Nast Magazines, *Women's Sports & Fitness*, IEZ Einkaufs Zentrum, TV Spielfilm, H. B. Fuller, West Publishing, Sony, Disney/ABC, and Paramount Pictures.

Andrei has photographed numerous personalities including Christian Slater, Marisa Tomei, Emilio Estevez, Trent Reznor, Marilyn Manson, and Kurt Cobain. His work has been been featured in galleries around the world, and he recently won The Klaus Schachtschneider Award for Excellence in Photography (Berlin), as well as the Marcel Richter Beautiful People Photography Award (Vienna). Recognized as one of the hottest young photographers in both Europe and Asia, he is a member of the Ilfo Pro Photographers' Association, and his biography appears in the 1998/1999 edition of *Who's Who in Media and Communications*.

Andrei wishes to dedicate his featured work in this book to the loving memory of Brook Johnson, talented make-up artist and dear friend. "You have made my work what it is today, and will continue to be an inspiration for many, many more shots to come."

Steven Andres—*www.stevenandres.com*

Based in Atlanta, Steven specializes in fashion, commercial, and fine-art photography. His work includes shooting for models, designers, musicians, and agencies in Atlanta and on location. His *Black & White Fine Art Projects* will be published this year in a European Fine Art Photography Anthology. He also has *Stock Photography* available in the U.S. and Japan. Steven Andres Photography, 1260 Foster St. Studio #34, Atlanta, Ga. 30318. (404) 352-1803. Email: *stevenandres@surfree.com*.

Erin Ashley

As a provider of "just right" photos for a modeling portfolio, Erin Ashley is top-notch because she knows all aspects of the business. She has worked as a model and an agent, and wrote and produced the instructional video *Working The Runway*, as well as running her own modeling agency! Erin Ashley gives clients the extra touch that agents love in each picture she creates. For your photo session call (805) 480–3333 (located in Southern California).

Stephen Clark—www.pbsclark.com

Located in Monticello, New York, Stephen is a fashion photographer for all your photographic needs worldwide. He specializes in editorial fashion but is also available for commercial/lifestyle, product, ad work, and model development. To book Stephen for your next assignment you may contact him directly or through his Artist Representative at his photo rep's page on the Web site. Please email any questions, booking information, rate sheets, or bids to *mjpart@pacificbell.net.*

Tom Farrington—www.webcom.com/tomkat

Based in San Diego, Tom has been widely published in international rock music and classic auto racing magazines. He also spent ten years as an entertainment photographer in L.A. for SIPA. He is currently expanding his work into the fashion/fine art venue.

Bradley Herlein—www.model-light.com

Bradley C. Herlein is the owner and photographer of model-light.com, a photo studio specializing in fashion, portfolio, and fine-art work. He is located in the Kansas City area. Other samples of his work can be viewed at his Web site, or you can contact him at *model-light@hotmail.com.*

Jorgen Hornsten-Gran

Jorgen Hornsten–Gran is an internationally working photographer located in southern Sweden. He is concentrating on, and caring for, people in different environments and situations in daily life as well as commercial, editorial and fashion. Jorgen is also the initiator and owner of Sofia Fotografer (*http://www.sofiafoto.nu*).

Gary Jones—www.nacs.net/~gjones

Based in Ravenna, Ohio, Gary is a fashion photographer specializing in commercial/lifestyle, ad work, and editorial fashion. He also does limited model development.

Harry Lang—www.harrylangphotography.com

Working out of Los Angeles, Harry's versatile style has been described as "edgy, high fashion, yet clean." His approach to fashion photography is to prompt models to exude an emotion that allows the viewer to gaze into the picture in a way that inspires them to react. With each shoot, he attempts something different, and consistently brings new ideas and creativity to every project. This ability enables any client—whether a model, magazine, or ad agency—to achieve top quality work with a dedicated and passionate photographer. Harry's specialties include fashion, editorial, commercial, and portrait photography. "When I'm working with a model, I try to bring out something inside of him or her, something that can communicate with the viewer—an emotion, a feeling, or a moment stopped in time . . . this is something I think separates my work, it's a little bit of myself, and that's what gives it a unique look." For further information on rates please send an e-mail (address at Web site) or call (323) 349–9705.

Chris Lawrence—www.clics-online.com

A professional freelance photographer based in the San Francisco Bay area, Chris has always been fascinated with cameras and photography. From a very early age, he experimented with pinhole cameras and solargrams. His first real photography job was shooting for a local portrait studio, and he continued portraiture work for a studio in Sacramento while attending UC Davis. "It was in the studio where I learned the physics of light and how to photograph people." Since then, he has enjoyed many exciting photographic assignments ranging from commercial product work to travel brochures. Chris is now focusing on the fashion/glamour side of the industry.

Bill Lemon—www.billlemon.com

Bill Lemon started his photography career in 1981 and has shot assignments for many large companies and top publications including Chevron, Mervyns, Marin Apparel Co., Alpha Vista Inc., Shutterbug, Napa Valley Appellation, Studio Photography, Photography Information Council, and California State Parks. His passion for fashion and beauty is evident in his work, as is his ability to capture the essence of the product, subject, and atmosphere all in one shot. Between conducting local workshops on fashion and glamour, Bill is busy photographing everything from engine parts, jewelry, and dinnerware to fashion layouts. He also has a new book on black-and-white glamour photography. For more information about his book or work, see his Web site.

D. Brian Nelson—*www.fotog.net*

Based in San Diego, California, and traveling extensively, D. Brian produces hard, avant, edgy, and powerful images depicting women and men of strength and emotion. D. specializes in editorial fashion assignments, figure with fashion styling, and anything else that strikes his fancy. Although he has been in and out of the fashion photography business for about twelve years, he is now making photographs for self-expression. His work can be seen publicly at his Web site and in an occasional gallery in San Diego.

Johnny Olsen—*www.johnyolsen.com*

A professional photographer for a decade, Johnny attended New York's School of Visual Arts, and worked with many talented and creative professionals. His most memorable moments shooting were spent on a three-month cross-country trip, photographing the National Parks of the western United States. He has photographed for modeling agencies in New York, Los Angeles, and San Diego, and clients across the country. He specializes in editorial fashion, commercial, and theatrical headshots using *only* natural lighting. In addition to photography, Johnny also operates a successful digital imaging business, which includes Web site design. Johnny Olsen Photography is located at 15136 Nordhoff St., North Hills, CA 91343. He says of his work: "The most important part of a good photo shoot is the chemistry between the photographer and the model. It is my job to make him/her feel comfortable. In all of my images, there is truly a relaxed feel. This makes the difference between good pictures and great pictures."

Jason Perkins—*http://users.abac.com/dbnelson/perk13*

Jason is new at fashion photography and aspires to shoot beauty as true to the human experience as possible. His plans are to shoot in terms of storyboards portraying lifestyles of the fashions in natural settings.

Karim Ramzi—www.karimramzi.com

Born in 1961 in Marrakech, Morocco, into a diplomatic family, Karim attended high school in Morocco and then the Royal College in Rabat, where King Mohammed VI was one of his fellow students. He graduated as one of the top five students in the country. He speaks Berber, French, Arabic, English, and Spanish. Post-graduate education at Ottawa University was in Political Science and Communication, while working for the French channel of the Moroccan radio as a show host and producer of a rock show, broadcasting his programs from Canada through the studios of CBC International. After a year as a reporter for *Charlatan* newsmagazine, he pursued a long-held interest in photography and became the paper's photo editor.

For over a decade, Karim has captured memorable images of both professional models and celebrities. He is commissioned on a regular basis to photograph the royal families of Saudi Arabia, Jordan, and Morocco, as well as other personalities around the world. He is one of the leading photographers in the Arab world and operates in Europe, the United States, the Middle East and occasionally in South East Asia. His successful one-man exhibitions have been in both Morocco (1988) and Saudi Arabia (1990); his photos were part of a joint exhibition in Tipasa, Algeria (1990). Entirely self-taught in photography, he readily acknowledges the influence and impact of others. While studying in Canada he met with the grand master of portrait photography, Yousuf Karsh, with whom he shared a mutual admiration. "He gave me a lot of invaluable tips," says Karim. "He knew every trick in the book. Neither of us had the doubt that one day he would do my portrait and I would do his." Karim also recognizes the influence of Alexey Brodovich, the late great graphic designer and art director of Harper's Bazaar in the forties.

Karim maintains that the fashion picture "is of the artificial and yet one seeks to show the whole aesthetic nature of the person wearing the clothes. A fashion photograph can be many things; it is a social phenomenon and it is an indication of sociology, it is a document of fashion since it can be a signal and a symbol of class, education, taste, and conformity or revolt. I think that the challenge in fashion photography is to see the fashion model as a human being and not only as a mannequin. I don't think there are any secrets in photography. To reach a certain standard one must take into consideration a series of factors including a reliable knowledge of the various photographic techniques, the problems they can cause and how to solve them, an eye well educated in aesthetics, a wide–ranging general knowledge and, above all, an astute ability to communicate with that which we photograph and that which surrounds us."

Karim resides in Paris, France, with his wife Naima and their daughter Sarah. He travels worldwide to capture images of personalities in their preferred venues.

Andrew Richard—www.canvas42.com

Andrew Richard is a New York–based fashion photographer and photo-journalist. His work can be seen in many publications both domestically and internationally. Andrew can be contacted by email at *info@canvas42.com* or by phone at (516) 791–4191.

Dr. Wood—www.drwood.com

Besides having a unique processing patent for film, Dr. Wood specializes in portrait editorial, actor headshots, editorial and commercial fashion, and model portfolio development. The Dr. Wood Foto Studio is located in the historic Santa Fe, which has been a part of downtown Los Angeles' historic landscape since 1923. Once the tallest building in LA, this eleven-story marvel was originally built as the main headquarters for the Santa Fe Railroad. To contact Dr. Wood for bookings, appointments, and directions, write 560 South Main St., Los Angeles, CA 90013, phone (213) 488-3453 or e-mail *drwood@drwood.com.*

Artists

Maria Vasseur is a graduate of Ventura College, with an A.S. in Fashion Design and Merchandising. She is currently studying Fine Art at College of the Canyons in Southern California.

Nicole Nolasco is a recent high school graduate. She is also a Fine Art student at College of the Canyons.

Glossary of Modeling and Related Terms

8 × 10 A photograph that is 8" × 10" in size. This generally refers to a headshot of the model.

Advance Money paid before the completion of a job that is later deducted from the model's pay. Sometimes advances are given to cover modeling expenses, testing, portfolio costs, and other expenses.

AFTRA A union for television performers called the American Federation of Television and Radio Artists.

Agency A company that serves as an employment agency to promote a model, set up appointments or "go-sees," schedule bookings, and negotiate fees or contracts for models for a percentage of the amount the model is paid for assignments.

Agent An individual who works for an agency who negotiates and books jobs for the model.

Beauty shot A headshot that emphasizes the model's face, hair, and makeup.

Book (1) The model's portfolio or the agency's book, which contain pictures, ads, covers, and tear sheets of the models whom the agency represents. (2) The assignment of a model for a specific job, also known as a "booking."

Booker Same as agent.

Booking A job that has been booked or confirmed for the model.

Booking out When the model blocks out time from his/her schedule, indicating dates and times the model will not be available to work.

Callback When a model is called back in to see a client. Similar to a second interview.

Casting The process of selecting a model for an assignment (television commercial, fashion show, print work, etc.).

Cattle call Refers to a lot of models competing for the job at the same time at a casting.

Character model A model who is neither a fashion– nor catalog–type model, but one who exhibits a variety of "character" looks, like an actor playing minor roles in a film, TV show, or stage play.

Chart A tracking system agencies use to manage time for their models.

Client The company or entity hiring the model.

Collection Various styles of clothing created by a designer(s).

Commentary Primarily used at fashion shows, commentary is the script or description of what is being shown.

Commentator The individual who speaks at a fashion show, describing and commenting on the fashions.

Commercial look A look that is common and appealing to a wide variety of consumers. A commercial model is usually one who models consumer products.

Commission The fee paid to the model's agent. This fee is a percentage of the model's earnings and is taken from the amount the client pays. The standard commission rate is 20 percent.

Composite A card or photo sheet of the model's photographs or tear sheets, generally including a variety of shots (headshot, swimwear, glamorous, etc.). The composite is the model's calling card or business card. It will also include the agency name, contact information, as well as the model's statistics (such as height, weight, and size).

Contact sheet A sheet (or photograph) of negatives as processed from a photo shoot. Usually 8" × 10", it contains the sequence of shots as processed from a roll of film. One usually views these images with a magnifying glass (also called a *loupe*). These are used to select the best photographs from a shoot.

Contract A legal agreement between the model and his/her agency, photographer, or client.

Convention/trade show Models are often used in trade shows and conventions to help attract attention to displays, to "meet and greet" prospective customers, or to demonstrate a product.

Day rate The daily rate the client pays to book a model. Usually this is for an eight-hour period of time.

Dresser The person who fits the model into wardrobe.

Editorial The section of a magazines that is devoted to doing a "fashion story" and is not tied into advertising. Most major magazines feature a fashion editorial section each month.

Fitting An appointment to make sure the model's clothing fits properly before a shoot or show. The term can also apply to models who work with designers to make sure their designs are fitting properly.

Freelance A self-promoting model who works on her own without agency representation.

Glamour Anything from modeling an elegant evening gown to posing nude. The term also refers to producing a glamorous headshot or an advertisement for display on cards, calendars, posters, billboards, magazines, etc.

Go-see A model's appointment to "go see" a client.

Head sheet An agency's marketing material used to promote its models, which is usually a poster with model's headshot and statistics.

Headshot A close-up photograph of the model that only includes the head and shoulders.

High fashion Usually refers to showing or modeling designer clothes or top-of-the-line accessories, cosmetics, or products. This is the highest paid and most well-known type of modeling.

Loupe A small, hand-held magnifying device used to view contact sheets.

Model release A contract that releases the model's rights to the photographs taken at the stated session. This contract is signed by the model to give his/her permission to use the photographs from a session or shoot.

Open call The period of time when agencies will see prospective models without an appointment.

Photographer release A contract signed by the photographer that gives the model permission to use the photographs taken during a particular sitting.

Plus-size A model who wears a larger size than conventional, or straight-size, models—usually a size twelve and up.

Portfolio A model's marketing materials. Also known as his/her "book," a portfolio is comprised of photographs or tear sheets that show the model's versatility, style, and photogenic quality.

Résumé A model's résumé specifically includes his/her education, experience, and statistics.

Runway A raised, stagelike platform that is about four feet wide and runs down the center of a room.

Runway model A model who works in fashion shows.

Shoot A photo session.

Shooting A session where a model poses for a photographer.

Stylist A professional who works on a photo shoot or runway show and provides props, accessories, and/or clothing.

Tear Sheet Pages of publications that show the model's image. These sheets are "torn" or removed from the publication and can include advertisements, magazine covers, editorial, or catalog work. Tear sheets go in the model's portfolio.

Tentative Usually referred to as a "tentative booking," this is a booking that has been placed on hold. The model's time is reserved, yet the booking has not been confirmed.

Test shoot A photographic session in which a model works with a photographer with the intent of creating a new idea and enhancing his/her portfolio. Usually, the model will pay for the cost of film or share developing costs only. Both the model and photographer should sign releases before the session.

Voucher A document supplied by the agency that stipulates the agreement between the client and model. It contains usage and billing information, the model's rates, and serves as a release for the model.

ZED Card See "composite card."

Index

Page numbers appear in italic for illustrations.

Accountants, 167–168
acting, 31, 34, 35, 40, 176, 227
Adair, Leslie, 49, 72
Adams, Jenni, 28
advance, defined, 245
advertising, 15–16
  acting-related, 31
  career in, 181
  commercial print modeling, 12
  international modeling for, 150–55
  responding to, 130–131
  small-town opportunities in, 76
African-American models, 5
AFTRA (American Federation of Television and Radio
      Artists), 236, 245
age, 39–40, 45
agencies, 85–96, 207–208, 224
  boutique, 81, 89
  contacting, 208
  at conventions, 203
  defined, 245
  directories for, 208
  Elite L.A., 93, 96
  Elite Model Management, 2
  expenses, model, 95–96
  Ford Modeling Agency, 35, 38, 192, xv
  fraudulent, 137
  Funny Face agency, 33
  Go International Model Management, 76–77
  housing provided by, 91, 92, 141–142, 145

international, 150, 214–224
John Robert Powers, 2
in major cities, 85–86
Model Management International (MMI), 76, 154
Model's Guild, The, 80
Models Mart, 77–78
mother, 87, 92, 151, 208
new faces division of, 91
new models, finding, 93–94
online, 158
parents on, advice for, 184–185
personnel at, 87–88, 90
promotion of models, 93
relocation provided by, 91–92
test board of, 91
travel provided by, 91–92
Ugly agency, 33
in the United States, 208–213
Web sites, 234–235
Wilhelmina agency, 35, 94
See also agency, finding the right; commissions;
      contracts; model management companies;
      model's apartments
agency, finding the right, 75–84
  in an average-size city, 77
  interviewing for, 80, 82
  in major markets, 77–78
  in a small town, 75–77
  tips for, 78–82
  unknown agencies, researching, 80, 83, 96, 133,

134–135
See also agencies; model management companies
agent(s), 87–88
    career as, 175–177
    defined, 245
    foreign, 88
    independent modeling without, 161–165
    relationship with, 88–89
    for success in modeling, 160
Alexis, Kim, 65
All That Jazz, 26
ambition, 46
apartments, model's. *See* model's apartments
appearance. *See* physical requirements
artists, 244
    See also Nolasco, Nicole; Vasseur, Maria
artist's representative/agent, career as, 181
Asian markets, 33, 50, 87, 150, 154–155, 185, 215,
    224
    See also markets
Asian models, 5
attitude, 46, 126
attributes for success. *See* success, attributes for
August, Michele, 116
Australia, 150–151, 214
Averill, Stephanie, 14, 49

Beauty shot, defined, 245
Beekman Hotel, 143
benefits, of modeling, 58
Bennett, Linda, 205
Better Business Bureau, 130, 139, 200
Big Beauties & Little Women, xiv
body care, 61–62
book cover modeling, 35
book, defined, 246
booker(s), 87, 176–177, 188, 246
booking, defined, 246
booking out, defined, 246
bookings, 115–126
    attitude for, 126
    first, 116
    forms for, 119–120, 121–122
    preparing for, 116–117
    professionalism for, 124–125
    rates for, 117–119
    scheduling, 119–120
    secondary, 121
    supplies for, 123–124
    tentative, 121
    test, 121
    wardrobe for, 124
books, 59, 224–226, 227
boutique agencies, 81, 89
Bredemeier, Kenneth, 133
broadcasting, career in, 181
Bureau of Consumer Protection Offices of Consumer and
    Business Education, 139
business, of modeling, 167–173
    budgeting, 1713–172
    See also contracts; Model's Guild, The; taxes
"buyout" fee, 117

Callbacks, 115, 202, 246
careers, in modeling-related industries, 175–182
    acting, 176
    advertising, 181
    agent/booker, 176–177
    artist's representative/agent, 181
    broadcasting, 181

    fashion designer, 177
    fashion stylist, 178
    hairstylist, 180
    magazine editors, 178
    makeup artist, 178–180
    photographer, 177
    public relations, 181–182
    set designer, 182
    stylist, 180
    writers, fashion, 178
Carmelite Sisters residence, 144
Casablanca, John, 2
casting, 73, 115, 246
catalog modeling, 12–15, 150–52, 154, 155
cattle call, defined, 246
Catwalk: Inside the World of the Supermodels (Morris),
    22
Centro Maria Residence, 145
change, in modeling, 5, 189
    See also trends
Chan, Kwok Kan, 48, 49, 54, 89
chaperones, 111, 130, 142, 163, 165, 188–189
character models, 40, 246
chart, defined, 246
"Chemical & Engineering News," 5
child models, 38–39, 131, 191–193
    See also parents, advice for
client, defined, 246
clothes. *See* wardrobe
Codner, Shannon Marie, 162–163, *163*, 164
collection, defined, 246
commentary, defined, 246
commentator, defined, 246
commercial look, defined, 246
commercial print modeling, defined, 12
commissions, 82, 86, 92, 151, 155, 173, 246
    See also income; rates
communication, 46–47
competition, 47, 58
composite cards
    agency on, working with, 88, 91, 93, 95
    for child models, 192
    at conventions, 204
    defined, 246
    for hairstylists, 180
    for independent modeling, 162
    on Internet, 99
    for makeup artists, 179
    resources, 229
    supply of, 108, 172
computer software, 69–70
confidence, 48
consumer protection, 133, 139, 231
Consumer Response Center, 139
contact sheets, 101, 102, 110, 246–247
contests, 94, 231, xiii
    See also conventions
contracts, 82, 83, 86, 92, 173
    defined, 247
    exclusive agreements, 15, 121
    parents on, advice for, 187
    scam, 128, 133, 137
    trial periods, 173
conventions, 94, 131, 201–206
    defined, 247
    Modeling Association of America International, Inc.
        (MAAI), 205
    Model Search America (MSA), *202*, 202–205
    New York Model Contracts, 205
    rip-offs at, 206

scams at, 137–139, 206
cosmetics, 15, 231
    See also makeup
Cosmopolitan, 7
"Cosmopolitan Virtual Makeover," 70
costs, modeling, 2, 95–96
        budgeting for, 171–172
        for children, 39
        international, 153, 154, 155
        for photography, 110
        for portfolios, 108–109
        tax-deductible, 169–170
        for training, 83
        See also money management
Crawford, Cindy, 81, 160
criticism, 48
    See also rejection

Day rate, defined, 247
Dell'Orefice, Carmen, 39
Denmark, 155
dental care, 44, 65
determination, 49
DICE, 229
diet, 72–73
digital imaging, 8, 181, 229, 242
directories, 226
discipline, 49
domain name, 165
dresser, defined, 247
drugs, 53–54, 136–137, 191

Easy Exotic: A Model's Low-Fat Recipes from Around the
        World (Lakshmi), 53
E! Channel, 5, 21
editor, career as, 178
editorial print
        careers in, 178
        defined, 247
        international modeling, 150, 151, 153, 154, 155
        modeling, 11–12
Edmonds, Shailah, 22
education, 54, 133, 188, 192–193, 233
8X10, defined, 245
Elite L.A., 37, 43, 85, 91, 94, 185, 186
Elite Model Management, 2
Elle, 26
Emme, 5
energy, 49–50
England, 151, 215–217
Esch, Natasha, 19
Essence, 94
exclusive agreements, 15, 121
    See also contracts
exercise, 72, 73
exfoliation, 60–61

Face, 44, 103
fashion
        books on, 227
        careers, 178
        designer, career as, 177
        resources, 231–232
        See also careers, in modeling-related industries
Fashion Emergency, 5
Fashion Institute of Technology, 145
"Fashion Week" (Germany), 153
Federal Trade Commission, 133, 139
feet, 65
film modeling, 31

Fin, Oja, 80
fit modeling, 27
fitting, defined, 247
flexibility, 6–7, 50, 120, 132–133
Ford Modeling Agency, 29, 35, 38, 80–81, 85, 181,
        185, 192, xv
France, 151–152, 217–222
fraud. *See* scams, avoiding
freelance, defined, 247
Frenchway Travel Agency, The, 145
full-figure models. *See* plus-size modeling
Funny Face agency, 33
future, planning for, 7, 54

Gens, Laura, 16–17
Georget, Susan, 35–36
Germany, 152–153, 222–223
glamour modeling, 18–20, 247
glossary, 245–248
Go International Model Management, 76–77
go-sees, 73, 88, 92, 115, 197, 247
Gramercy Park Hotel, 143
Greece, 153
grooming, 59
grunge trend, 5

Hair, 44, 69–70, 120, 180
head sheet, 93, 247
headshot, defined, 247
health, 70
health insurance, 170
height, 43–44
        international modeling requirements for, 150–55
high-fashion modeling, 11, 247
Hispanic models, 5
hold, 121
homesickness, 146, 190–191
H.O.P.E. (Helping Others to Perform with Excellence), 7
hotels, in New York City, 143
        See also model's apartments; residences, in New
            York City
housing. *See* model's apartments
How to Be a Successful Runway Model (Edmonds), 22
Hutton, Lauren, 81

Image, 58–59, 106–107
income, 1–2, 9–10
        advertising modeling, 15
        catalog modeling, 13, 14
        for character models, 40
        from child modeling, 193
        earned by top models, 1–2
        film modeling, 31
        fit modeling, 27
        full-figure models, 36
        for independent modeling, 163
        male model, 37
        parts modeling, 16
        promotional modeling, 30
        residual payments, 117
        runway modeling, 20
        from scams, 132
        specialty modeling, 16
        supplementing, 170–171
        television modeling, 31
        See also commissions; rates
independence, 50–51
independent contractor, model as, 96, 167, 168, 193
independent modeling, 161–165, 163–164
informal modeling, 30

insurance, 96, 170
International House, 145
international modeling, 149–156
    agencies, 150, 214–224
    agent relationship, 88
    countries for, 150–156
    International Freelance Models Organization (IFMO), 233
    magazines, 12
    markets, 11–12, 33, 35, 76–77, 92, 152
    model management companies, 86–87
    nudity in Europe, attitudes toward, 20
    school placement for, modeling, 197
    transportation for, 151, 152, 153, 155, 156
    travel, 92, 145–148
    types of, 150–55
    See also Asian markets
Internet, 7–8, 54, 57–58, 59, 157–165
    agencies online, 158
    bulletin boards, 162
    chat sites, 158–159
    composites on, 99
    contest information, 94
    domain name, 165
    e-mail, 162
    forums, 158–159
    independent modeling on, 161–165
    newsgroups, 158–159, 162
    pornographic sites, 159
    portfolios on, 99
    scams, information to avoid, 134–135, 139, 158
    search engines, 159
    See also computer software; Web site(s)
interviews, agency, 80, 81
Italy, 153–154, 223–224

J apan, 154–155, 224
jealousy, 49
Joe's, 19
John Robert Powers, 2

K atherine House, 144
Klein, Calvin, 11

L akshmi, Padma, 51
large-size modeling. See plus-size modeling
LeBook, 151–153
Lee, Karen, 91
lingerie models, 19
local modeling, 4, 76
locations for modeling, major-city, 4
Loews New York Hotel, 143
Lombardy Hotel, 143
longevity in modeling, 7, 14–15, 16, 33, 36, 37, 49
Long, Sherrie, 179, 179–180
Los Angeles Times Magazine, 2, 107
loupe, 101, 247
Luca, Luca, 26

M ackie, Bob, 26
MacPherson, Elle, 2, 107
Madison Towers Hotel, 144
magazines, 12, 59, 99, 153, 176, 178, 233
makeup
    advice, 103–104
    applying, 104–106
    artist, career as, 178–180
    for bookings, 120
    books on, 102, 226–227
    computer software for, 69–70

as expense, 95
in Germany, 153
kit, 66–67
learning to contour, 104–105
lessons, 59, 66
for photography, 102–106
products/lessons, resources for, 228
skills, 67–69
in Switzerland, 156
tools, 103
    See also cosmetics
Makeup For Ever Professional, 66, 103, 228
male models, 36–37
managing mother agency, 92
manicures, 63–64, 103
mannequin modeling, 27
Marie, Joanna, 48
Marilyn, Inc., 48, 49, 54, 89
markets, 4
    average-size city, 77
    international, 11–12, 33, 35, 76–77, 92, 152
    major, 77–78, 85
    small, 75–77, 110, 134
    See also Asian markets
Markle Residence, The, 144
massage, 61–62
Matheson, Eve, 150
mature models, 39–40
McDonald, Julian, 26
meditation, 71
messengers, 95
Mode, 5, 35, 94
model, defined, 2
Modeling Association of America International, Inc. (MAAI), 205
Modeling Handbook, The (Matheson), 150
modeling, types of, 9–31
    advertising, 15–16, 31
    bookcover, 35
    catalog, 12–15, 150, 151, 152, 154, 155
    commercial print, 12
    editorial print, 11–12, 150, 151, 153, 154, 155, 178, 247
    film, 31
    fit, 27
    glamour, 18–20, 247
    high-fashion, 11
    informal, 30
    parts, 16–18, 35
    print, 10–16
    promotional, 29–31
    runway, 20–27, 151, 153, 248
    showroom, 27–29
    specialty, 16–18
    tea-room, 30
    television, 31, 117, 155
    See also models, types of
model management companies, 76–77, 86–87, 94, 161, 234–235
    See also agencies
Model Management International (MMI), 76, 154
Model Manual, The (Morris), 33–34
model releases, 111–114, 122, 247
    See also photography
model's apartments, 91, 92, 142, 145
    See also residences, in New York City
model's bag, 95, 116, 123–124
Model Search America (MSA), 202, 202–205
Model's Guild, The, 80, 170, 208
Model's Mart, 77–78, 108, 208

models, types of, 33–40
   character, 40, 246
   child, 38–39, 131, 191–193
   male, 36–37
   mature, 39–40
   petites, 34–35
   plus-size, 5, 35–36, 94, 248
   real people, 15–16, 40
   swimwear, 19
   teen, 36–38, 183–184, 185–191
   See also modeling, types of
Mogull, F. David, 202
moisturizer, 61, 104
money management, 49–50
   with agencies, 95–96
   budgeting, 171–172
   in Italy, 154
   parents on, advice for, 189–190, 193
   resources, 53
   savings, 172, 190, 193
   when traveling, 148
Morris, Sandra, 22, 33–34
Moss, Kate, 11, 19
mother agency, 87, 92, 151, 208
Mullins, Aimee, 6–7

Nail care, 63–65
Nancy Bounds Studios, Inc., 138–139, 196–197
newsgroups, 230
New York
   agencies in, 80, 211–213
   hotels in, 143
   industry standards, 43–45
   as main fashion market, 36, 95
   relocating to, 141–145
   residences in, 141–142, 144–145
New York Model Contracts, 205
Nolasco, Nicole, 60, 244
Norway, 155
nudity, 18–20, 129–130, 135–136
nutrition, 72–73
"NYC Taxi and Limousine Drivers Guide," 143

Open call, 79, 80, 93, 247
option, 121
organization, 51, 119–120
Overton, Mona, 76

Palumbo, Franca, 37
parents, advice for, 183–193
   on agencies, 184–185
   on career management, 186–188
   on child modeling, 191–193
   on coping with change, 189
   on education, 188, 192–193
   on happiness in modeling, 191
   on homesickness, 190–191
   on money management, 189–190, 193
   on rejection, 191
   on starting out, 185–186
   on teens in adult market, 183–184
   on travel, 188–189
   on trust, 185–186
Parkside Evangeline Residence, The, 144
parts modeling, 16–18, 35
passport, 145, 147, 148
patience, 50
pedicures, 65, 103
perseverance, 51–52
Persinger, Michele, 185

personality, 46, 52
Peter Glenn Publications, 208
Peterson, Danielle, 52
petite models, 34–35
photogenic quality, 45
photographers, 172
   Andrei, 47, 66, 98, 100–101, 237–238
   Andres, Steven, 238
   Ashley, Erin, 10, *184*, *187*, 238–239
   career as, *177*
   Clark, Stephen, *12*, *77*, *132*, *142*, 239
   Elgort, Arthur, 19
   Farrington, Tom, *70*, 240
   finding, 110, 165
   Flax, Jeff, *109*
   Herlein, Bradley Charles, *79*, 240
   Hornsten-Gran, Jorgen, *28*, *29*, 240
   Jones, Gary, *30*, 240
   Lang, Harry, *59*, *93*, 240–241
   Lawrence, Chris, *44*, *61*, *62*, 241
   from LeBook, 151–152
   Lemon, Bill, 14, *19*, 241
   Lewin, Gideon, 188
   for mature models, 40
   Nelson, D. Brian, *36*, *38*, *105*, *107*, *129*, 241–242
   Olsen, Johnny, *33*, *42*, *86*, 98–99, *99*, *116*, *121*, *171*, 242
   Patton, Chris, xii
   Perkins, Jason, *172* 242
   Peterson, Dan, *163*
   Petrucci, Luria, *47*, *159*, 159–160
   posing for, 99–102
   Ramzi, Karim, *17*, *18*, *20*, *58*, *64*, *68*, *98*, *100*, *146*, *147*, *150*, *152*, 242–243
   Richard, Andrew, *3*, *20*, *22*, *23*, *24*, 24–27, *25*, *26*, *39*, 244
   Ritts, Herb, 19
   in small-towns, 76
   Snaric, Martin, 22–23, xiv, xv
   testing with, 88, 91, 93, 95, 109–111, 151, 163, 197, 248
   Weber, Bruce, 19
   Web sites, 235–236
   Wood, Dr., *102*, 244
   working with, 47, 97–99
   Young, Kingmond, *179*
   See also photography
photography
   chaperones, 111
   for child models, 192
   computerized, 7–8
   at conventions, 204
   costs, 135
   makeup, 66, 102–106
   releases, model, 111–114, 122, 247, 248
   shoots, 49
   stock, 163
   submissions, 79–80, 94
   See also composite cards; photographers; portfolios; testings
physical requirements, 43–45
   appearance, flexibility in, 6–7
   in international modeling, 150–55
Pillard, Monique, 43, 45, 186
plus-size modeling, 5, 35–36, 94, 248
portfolios, 93, 107–111
   for agencies, 81, 83, 92, 93
   defined, 248
   as expense, 85, 95, 172

for hairstylists, 180
on Internet, 99
for makeup artists, 179
from modeling school, 197
photography for, 83, 88
in scams, 135
See also photographers; photography
posing, 99–102
poster, 93
posture, 44, 62–63
Preti, Pascal, 97
print modeling, 10–16
    advertising, 15–16
    catalog, 12–15
    commercial, 12
    editorial, 11–12
    high-fashion, 11
professionalism, 52–53, 124–125, 151, 152, 155
promotion, 93, 161–165
promotional books, 93
promotional modeling, 29–31
Proulx, Kristina, 154–155
pseudonym, for independent modeling, 162
public relations, 90, 181–182

Quick, Rebecca, 21

Rapid White Tooth Whitening System, 65
rates, 117–119
    See also commissions; income
recruiting models, 93–94
rejection, 53, 84, 191
    See also criticism
relocation, 91–92, 141–145
residences, in New York City, 141–145
    See also model's apartments
residual payments, 117
resources, 225–236
    books, 225–228, 229
    consumer protection, 231
    contests, 231
    cosmetics, 231
    digital services, 229
    fashion, 231–232
    forums, 230
    makeup products/lessons, 228
    newsgroups, 230
    supplies, modeling, 229
    videos, 228
    See also Internet; Web site(s)
résumé, defined (diacritical marks), 248
Robertson, Kathy, 76
Rose, Wendy, 38, 185, 192
Rudisill, Karl, 42, 50, 181
runway modeling, 20–27, 151, 153, 248
    Richard, Andrew, interview with, 24–27
    walking the walk, tips for, 21–23

Sacred Heart Residence, 145
Salvation Army, 144
Sassy, 37
scams, avoiding, 127–139
    advertisements, responding to, 130–131
    agencies, researching unknown, 134–135
    Attorney General's office, state, 139
    Better Business Bureau, 139
    for child models, 131
    on contracts, 137
    at conventions, 137–138, 206
    by examination of true potential, 134

Federal Trade Commission for, 133, 139
    fees, caution about, 133–134, 135
    flexibility of schedules in, 132–133
    instincts for, listening to, 128–130
    Internet, using, 134–135, 139, 158
    knowledge for, importance of, 127
    nudity cautions, 135–136
    salaries, beware of high, 132
    school cautions, modeling, 138–139
    scouts, understanding, 133–134
    substance abuse cautions, 136–137
    unprofessional behavior warnings, 135–136
Scandanavia, 155
schedules, 132–133, 155
Schiffer, Claudia, 19
schools, modeling, 77, 83, 96, 195–198
    cautions about, 138–139
    costs of, 198
    finding, 197–198
    fraudulent, 137
    investigating, 198
    legitimate, 138–139
    role-model, 196–197
scouting, 93–94, 133–134
Screen Actors Guild (SAG), 31
seasons. *See* timing
self-image, 58
set designer, career as, 182
Seventeen, 37
Sherry-Netherland Hotel, 143
Shiatsu, 62
shoot, defined, 248
shooting, defined, 248
Short, Charles, 94
Short-Term Housing, 145
showroom modeling, 27–29
Sirot, Ellen, 17
skin care, 44, 59, 60–61
sleep, 70
smoking, 73
Spain, 155
specialty modeling, 16–18
spokesmodels, 29, 235
stress, 70–71, 176
stylist, defined, 248
success, attributes for, 41–55
    ambition, 46
    attitude, 46, 126
    communication, 46–47
    competitive, 47
    criticism, ability to accept, 48
    determination, 49
    discipline, 49
    energy, 49–50
    flexibility, 50
    independence, 50–51
    interests, having other, 51
    jealousy, understanding, 50
    money management, 50–51
    motivation, 41–42
    organization, 51
    patience, 50
    perseverence, 51–52
    personality, 52
    physical, 43–45
    professionalism, 52–53
    rejection, handling, 53
    resources, having, 53
    strength, 53–54
    vision of the future, 54

weight management, 54
sunblock, 62, 103
Sweden, 155
swimwear models, 19
Switzerland, 155–156

Tanning products, self, 62
taxes, 96, 146, 151, 167, 168–170, 172, 193
"tea room" modeling, 30
tear sheets, 88, 93, 95, 99, 149, 153, 180, 248
technology, impact of, 7–8
Teen, 37
teen models, 36–38, 183–184, 185–191
     See also parents, advice for
television modeling, 117, 155
Ten-Eyck Troughton Residence, 145
tentative, defined, 248
test board, 91
testings, 88, 91, 93, 95, 109–111, 151
     with agencies, 121
     defined, 248
     for independent modeling, 163
     from modeling school, 197
timing, 5, 20
trade shows, defined, 247
training, 195–198
     See also schools, modeling
travel, 91–92, 141–148
     agents, 145
     for bookings, 117, 120
     expenses, 92, 96
     health insurance, 146
     homesickness, 146, 190–191
     insurance, 146
     international, 92, 145–148
     money management, 148
     parents on, advice for, 188–189
     passport, 145, 147, 148
     willingness to, importance of, 4
trends
     changing, 5–6, 43
     for character models, 40
     for child models, 38
     girl-next-door, 5
     grunge, 5
     heroin chic, 5
     studying fashion, 58
Turlington, Christy, 51

Ugly agency, 33, 217

Vando, David, 77–78
Vasseur, Maria, 71, 72, 118, 123, 124, 168, 244
Victoria's Secret, 13, 21
videos, 228
Village Voice, The, 19
vitamins, 72–73
Vogue, 12, 26, 35
voucher, 121–122, 248

Walk, model's, 21–23, xiv
Wall Street Journal, 21
wardrobe, 73, 74, 124, 172
Washington Post, 133
Weamer, Carole, 103
Web site(s), 229–236
     agencies, 8, 234–235
     America Models Promotions, 161
     American Federation of Television and Radio Artists
        (AFTRA), 235

Codner, Shannon Marie, 162, 164
consumer protection, 231
for contests, 94, 231
for cosmetics, 231
design of, 164, 242
Digicomps™, 235
education, 233–234
fashion, 231–232
Federal Trade Commission, 139
for forums, 230
Go International Model Management, 76
International Freelance Models Organization (IFMO),
     233
LeBook, 151–152
for magazines, 233
Modeling Association of America International, Inc.
     (MAAI), 205
for modeling information, 232
Modelling Association of Canada, The, 233
model management company, 234–235
Model Management International, 76
for models, 159–160, 233
Model Search America (MSA), 205
Model's Guild, The, 233
for newsgroups, 230
Petrucci, Luria, 159–160
photographer, 237–244
photographers, for finding, 165, 235–236
for scams, 134–135
Screen Actors Guild (SAG), 235
Spokesmodel International, LLC, 235
Victoria's Secret, 21
Webster's Dictionary, 2
weight management, 44, 54, 73
White, Brian, 37
Wilhelmina Guide to Modeling, The (Esch), 19
Wilhelmina International, Ltd., 28–29, 35, 36, 37, 85,
     94
workshops, 170
writer, career as fashion, 178

Yoga, 71, 72

ZED Card. *See* composite cards

Books from Allworth Press

Promoting Your Acting Career
by Glenn Alterman (softcover, 6 × 9, 224 pages, $18.95)

Creative Careers in Music
by Josquin des Pres and Mark Landsman (6 × 9, 288 pages, $18.95)

Sex Appeal: The Art of Allure in Graphic and Advertising Design *by Steve Heller* (softcover, 6¾ × 10, 288 pages, $18.95)

An Actor's Guide—Your First Year in Hollywood
by Michael Saint Nicholas (softcover, 6 × 9, 256 pages, $16.95)

Songwriter's and Musician's Guide to Nashville, Revised Edition *by Sherry Bond* (6 × 9, 224 pages, $18.95)

Creating Your Own Monologue
by Glenn Alterman (6 × 9, 192 pages, $14.95)

Booking and Tour Management for the Performing Arts
by Rena Shagan (softcover, 6 × 9, 272 pages, $19.95)

Money Secrets of the Rich and Famous
by Michael Reynard (hardcover, 6½ × 9½, 256 pages, $24.95)

Please write to request our free catalog. To order by credit card, call 1-800-491-2808 or send a check or money order to Allworth Press, 10 East 23rd Street, Suite 210, New York, NY 10010. Include $5 for shipping and handling for the first book ordered and $1 for each additional book. Ten dollars plus $1 for each additional book if ordering from Canada. New York State residents must add sales tax.

To see our complete catalog on the World Wide Web, or to order online, you can find us at *www.allworth.com*.